Tangled Expectations

By Cathy Asselin

Copyright © 2013 by Cathy Asselin
First Edition – May 2013

ISBN
978-1-4602-1309-4 (Hardcover)
978-1-4602-1310-0 (Paperback)
978-1-4602-1311-7 (eBook)

Produced by:

FriesenPress

Suite 300 – 852 Fort Street
Victoria, BC, Canada V8W 1H8

www.friesenpress.com

Distributed to the trade by The Ingram Book Company

Table of Contents

Life is what happens to you
when you're busy making other plans.
John Lennon

Dedication

For my parents, my brother and sister,

and all those dear, life-long friends

with whom I am blessed.

Apparently we did sign up for this.

You granted me the honour of being

part of your journeys

and you've hung in on mine.

Thank you.

This is a story about gifts and teachers,

those whose books, CDs, videos and webinars I purchased;

and for those who reach the top shelf in stores

for products I need.

Thank you.

This is a story about waking up.

To Dan and Kevin --

You changed my life.

Thank you.

Cass XO
Edmonton, Alberta
April, 2013

Introduction

As World War I was coming to an end, my grandfather travelled home to Canada on a troop ship from England. It was the height of the Spanish flu pandemic, which is estimated to have killed between twenty and forty million people worldwide. The soldiers on my grandfather's ship were sick and dying with the deadly illness and the crossing took three weeks. My grandfather never got sick. If illness is simply a matter of biology, then why didn't my grandfather get the Spanish flu when he was quarantined on a ship for three weeks that was filled with sick and dying soldiers?

My father never got the classic childhood diseases. Why didn't he get the mumps, measles or chickenpox?

How did I, a direct descendent of an immune system like that, develop an auto-immune disease like multiple sclerosis?

Segment 1 – End Beginning

The world is round

and the place which may seem like the end

may also be the beginning.

George Baker

They Come in All Shapes and Sizes

When I was little, thinking about what I would be when I was all grown up, never once did a wheelchair figure in my imaginings.

I was a secretary before we were called administrative assistants. I worked for a small but busy commercial real estate development company in Edmonton. On my lunch hour I quite often ran around the downtown core doing errands, some personal, some for the office. I would pick up something to eat back at my desk between answering phone calls, filling the photocopier with toner, and typing leases for our latest project.

After working for the company for six years, in the spring of 1994, I noticed that sometimes by the time I got back to my desk with a sandwich, my right foot would be sloppily hitting the floor slowing me down a bit. If I sat at my desk for about 10 minutes that weakness disappeared and I was up and running again. It was annoying but I didn't give it much thought. Maybe I just slightly pulled a muscle or something like that. And besides, it didn't happen every time I was out running errands.

This day, I had been doing my usual running around on my lunch hour. Actually, I hadn't been "running" anywhere. I was barely walking. I could go three blocks in one direction, turn around, and walk three blocks back before I had to sit down. Sit down or fall down. Six blocks round-trip. That was my max. The distance I was able to walk had gradually been getting shorter and shorter. Today, it had taken my entire lunch hour to do the six-block-round-trip. I was a few steps from the final intersection. My building was on the opposite corner. Two more steps. The green light turned yellow.

No.

One more step. The red hand -- Do Not Walk -- flashed on the signal box.

I can't. My legs are too tired. Please. I'm almost there.

The traffic light turned red.

No.

I stared at the glass doors of the office tower, focusing on my objective, when a panhandler walked into my line of sight. He was standing in front of the building asking people for change as they crossed the street from the other direction. They walked past him, opened the building doors and went inside. When there were no more people crossing the street from that direction he turned and looked at my corner. I saw him but I was looking behind him, focused on the building doors and silently giving myself a pep talk.

You can do it. You can get there. Get to the doors. Go to the elevators. Walk down the hall. Sit at your desk. You can do it.

The light changed and I stepped off the curb as carefully as I could. People hurried past me, trying to get back to their desks before the end of their lunch breaks. They hopped up on the opposite sidewalk, sidestepped the panhandler, pulled open the office tower doors and disappeared inside.

Cursing curbs, I steadied my balance and brought my second foot down to the pavement. One step at a time, one slow, unsteady step at a time I walked towards those doors. The flashing red hand was blinking at me from the signal box.

Do Not Walk. Do Not Walk. Clear the Intersection.

Please God, don't let me fall down. Please.

I took one step at a time and stared hard at those glass doors. The panhandler watched, waiting for me to get to the corner so he could ask for change.

Please don't make me stop. If I stop I'll fall down. Please. I can't right now.

The curb was in sight. With every ounce of strength I had left I got one foot up on the sidewalk.

Okay. Again.

I steadied myself and with a second massive effort I pulled up my second foot. I didn't catch my toe. I didn't fall down. *Yeah.*

I felt the whoosh of cars passing behind me as I stood on the edge of the curb. I probably looked like I'd had a little too much to drink at lunch. I could have used a celebratory drink right then but instead, I focused on those office tower doors and took a determined step towards sanctuary.

And then the panhandler opened the door for me. He didn't say a word and he didn't ask for change. Maybe he figured I was having a harder day than he was so he did the kindest thing anyone could have done for me at that moment - he opened that great, big, beautiful, shiny, glass door for me.

Somehow I got to the elevator and somehow I got back to my desk and that panhandler became a teacher with an eye-opening lesson for me. Not all angels are blonde with flowing robes and soft, white feathery wings. Sometimes they're more beautiful than that.

Another Curb

Later on in July, 1994, I had to have a hysterectomy to get rid of fibroid tumors. At my six-week checkup, I complained to the surgeon that I wasn't walking quite right. He said not to worry. I was forty-one years old and had just had major surgery. I was probably taking a little longer to recuperate. But in the next few months other things started to happen. In the grocery store, when I reached for a bottle of ketchup, my arm suddenly started to shake so that I didn't dare take the bottle off the shelf for fear of dropping it. Sometimes in the morning when I was having my shower and I was washing my hair, both of my arms would suddenly go numb and fall limp to my sides leaving the shampoo streaming down my face. After a few moments the strength would return to my arms and I would finish my shower. I didn't like that sensation at all.

Edmonton's river valley is gorgeous and when the weather was good I liked walking the trails along the river and in the ravines. As winter came on, I took to going to the Kinsmen Centre and walking on the indoor track. I would throw on my headset, put a cassette tape in the Walkman and start walking, inspired by a driving beat

– Annie Lennox – *walking on, walking on bro-ken glaaass*. But with each trip I made to the track, the more it felt like I was walking through water, pushing against the force of a strong current, and the water was rising.

One evening, I was at the Kinsman with a friend and instead of walking around the track I opted for riding a stationary bike. Riding the bike was no problem at all until I stopped and got off. I fell flat on the floor because my legs had given out. After a few minutes sitting on my rear end pretending that I had slipped, I managed to get to my feet. I went to the locker room to change for the drive home. My friend followed me in her car to make sure I got there all right. Because I had twenty minutes sitting in my car to rest while driving, when I got out of the car I was fine. I waved goodbye to her and walked up the steps to the door of my apartment building no problem.

Another friend and I decided to treat ourselves to a weekend in Banff. I enjoyed the hotel's spa area until I couldn't get out of the hot tub. I had been in the tub for about fifteen minutes when I decided to get out. I discovered I had no strength and couldn't get out on my own. That was scary. Other people had to pull me out and get me to a bench. I lay on the bench for a few minutes cooling off and then wobbled back to the hotel room. After another half hour of lying down and resting, I got up and got dressed for dinner. I walked into the hotel dining room wearing high heels, like nothing had happened.

I made an appointment with my GP to tell her about these incidents but from the exam we did she determined that nothing in particular was happening, nothing was wrong that she could see. The symptoms came and went. During the exam they weren't evident at all. Maybe it was a pinched nerve. Maybe I was crazy, I thought, and had just been imagining these things. We would just have to wait and see what happened next – if anything.

In January, 1995 I went back to the surgeon who had done my hysterectomy and asked him, "Did you leave something in there?"

I told him I still wasn't walking right and there were these other odd things that were happening. He asked a lot of questions and one of them was did anyone in my family have multiple sclerosis? I said 'no' and he suggested I make an appointment at the Back Institute to see if they could find something.

So off I went to the Back Institute, not expecting much but in the course of having all kinds of reflexes tested on me, suddenly the therapist excitedly identified a "positive Babinski".

A what?

He got another therapist to verify what he was seeing and then he got on the phone with my GP, the gynecologist who had done the hysterectomy and an orthopedic surgeon who cleared time on his schedule to see me at 8 a.m. the next morning.

Now that is the definition of scary - when a specialist clears space on his schedule at the beginning of the next day and puts a perfect stranger at the head of the line in front of other patients who have had appointments for weeks or months. First appointment the next morning I was going to be the perfect stranger who walks into the specialist's office and takes up his valuable time and attention ahead of everyone else sitting in that waiting room. I got to be first the next day because apparently there were a whole lot of bells and whistles and alarms associated with a reflex named Babinski.

Warning, warning, Will Robinson. Danger.

I left the Back Institute and wandered next door to an engineering company where a friend of mine worked. I was in the neighbourhood. Thought I'd drop by and say hi.

Don't want to go home.

How are the kids?

I think something bad is happening to me.

Did you see the game last night?

Yup, I'm just kind of hanging out, killing time until 8 a.m. tomorrow.

The Messenger

As arranged, at 8 a.m. the next morning I was in the orthopedic surgeon's office. He put me through my paces with a series of commands including stand on your toes, walk on your heels, close your eyes and touch your index finger to the end of your nose. His conclusion: I either had a brain tumor, a tumor on my spine or multiple sclerosis.

At 10:30 a.m. that morning I was in my GP's office with my parents listening to her suggestions for what my options were at that point. I could wait six to eight months to get an appointment for a public MRI. I could make arrangements for an MRI to be done privately. That could happen almost immediately but would be expensive. Or I could have a spinal tap.

A spinal tap? Are you insane? This cannot be happening to me.

I went back to the orthopedic surgeon and told him I had decided to have the private MRI. Without hesitation, he got on the phone with the clinic. He wanted four sections photographed from the top of my head to the tip of my tailbone. How much would that cost he wanted to know. 'No,' he said into the phone. They could do better

9

than that. He sent them enough business. They should give me a deal. He arm-wrestled their price to almost half the figure they originally quoted him and God bless my parents, they paid for it. I didn't have that kind of money and I didn't want to wait six to eight months to find out what was wrong with me.

The appointment for the private MRI happened within a couple of days. The letters MRI stand for magnetic resonance imaging but I didn't know what that meant. It turns out there are magnets banging around the metal tube I was lying in. When a section of my spine was being photographed, the magnets banged. Sometimes the banging sounded low and slow and sometimes it sounded high and fast. But it was always loud. I hadn't been expecting all that banging. Neither was I expecting the headset and microphone that allowed me to communicate with the technician in the booth and listen to music between the episodic banging.

After each of the four segments was photographed, I could get out of the metal tube and take a look at the technician's screen and see my body's skeleton. There were my bones in black and white. Odd, but fascinating. Then it was back to the tubular DJ to have my ears pummeled by banging magnets between listening to Top 40 hits.

A couple of days later, the gynecologist who had done my hysterectomy phoned me at work. He asked if anybody had called to give me the results of the MRI. I said no. The MRI clinic hadn't called and neither had the orthopedic surgeon or my GP. He asked if I was sitting down. I said yes. Then he said, "You have multiple sclerosis." After a few silent moments he said, "I have one thing to say to you." There was another pause and then with gusto he said, *"Remission."*

I had completed my medical investigation in an orderly fashion from calling my GP about my sloppy right foot to getting an MRI done. I got the answer March 2, 1995. I had primary progressive multiple sclerosis. It was a Thursday.

On Friday morning my uncle Bill died. He was my father's only sibling and older brother. I went to work, called the local chapter of the MS Society and asked them for some information. A couple of hours later I received a package for the "newly diagnosed". The first piece of paper on the top of the stack I pulled out of the envelope was pink. At the top of the pink page in black, block lettering about an inch high was the word 'pain'. I shoved the stack of papers back into the envelope and tossed it into my bottom desk drawer. I should have thrown it away. Instead, I gradually started to fall apart.

And the Shoreline Disappeared

When I came up for air after that week from hell that included my uncle's funeral in Calgary, the next date on my agenda was an appointment with a neurologist that was arranged for me once I had the diagnosis. At the time, either there weren't a lot of neurologists in the city or he was the only one who was interested in MS because it seemed that anybody who had a diagnosis of multiple sclerosis was sent to see this doctor. I thought he would be a man of information who would tell me everything I needed to know about multiple sclerosis and have a game plan for how we were going to deal with it and get better. I was wrong.

He asked me to do the same sort of exercises that the orthopedic surgeon had asked me to do so he could get an idea of where I was at physically – stand on my toes, walk on my heels, close my eyes and touch the end of my nose with the tip of my index finger. I got through all of that easily enough and then he took out an x-ray sheet and put it on the lighted glass panel for me to see.

The x-ray film showed a series of brain images. He said, "Do you see those little white spots in the various brains?" I said I did and he took the x-ray down. He slipped another x-ray on the lighted panel. It was the same sort of thing -- a series of brain images on the one piece of film. He said, "Do you see the spots in the brains on this x-ray? They're bigger." I said I did and he took that x-ray down.

He slipped a third x-ray on the panel. With a pencil he pointed out the white matter in each of the brains. "You see where all the spots are bigger and they've joined together?" I said yes. Then he said, "You have little spots." And he took the third x-ray off the panel. I asked if the first x-ray showing the brains with the little white spots were pictures of my brain from the MRI I had done. He said no.

If you're waiting for me to report that he said something else, so was I but there was nothing. He just said no.

He took me into another office where a woman sat behind a desk. He said she would be my contact from now on and he left the room. I sat down and she took out a business card. On the back she wrote a telephone number and handed it to me saying that was the number to call when I was ready to get my wheelchair. I was still able to walk, not well, but I was able to walk and this woman hands me her business card with a phone number handwritten on the back and says this is where I'm supposed to call when I want my wheelchair.

This was not encouraging.

She said she would be the person to call if I had any questions or needed any help with "things". Did this mean the good doctor was no longer going to be involved with my case now that he had exhausted his show-and-tell x-ray demonstration?

The woman told me to see the receptionist who would line up the date for my annual appointment with the good doctor. I went to the reception desk and the appointment secretary very efficiently picked out a date one year hence when I would come back for my annual checkup. I told her I had a GP who I had annual checkups with and we could arrange to have those results sent to the neurologist's office. The appointment secretary corrected me with a tinge of haughtiness. Oh no, I was informed, from now on I would have all my annual checkups done by the good doctor and they would copy my GP on test results. Part of my annual checkup, I was informed, would include a spinal tap. An annual spinal tap? Yes.

As I was walking out of the waiting room there was a man in a wheelchair who looked to be a couple of years older than me sitting beside a woman I assumed was his wife. He was waiting to see the good doctor. Our eyes met and for a moment I was overwhelmed with the urge to take hold of his wheelchair, push him out to the elevators and tell him to get out of there as fast as he could. But I walked by him and made my own way to the elevators so I could get out of there myself. I walked across the parking lot to my car and after I got inside I just sat there for a few minutes. Then in the privacy of my car I said out loud, *"Dear God, I don't know how I'm going to do this but I'm not going to do that."*

That was the moment I stepped off the edge and away from conventional western medicine and entered the "alternative" world. In that moment, I didn't know that's what I was doing. I didn't know there were such things as "alternative modalities". All I knew in that moment was that there *had to be something else.* I didn't completely abandon conventional western medicine but from where I sat that afternoon, it was going to take a whole lot of answers to questions I didn't even know I had before I went sailing into another neurologist's office or any other doctor's office for that matter. From now on my guard would be way up.

Sitting in my car telling God out loud I wasn't going to do "that", implying that He'd best come up with something else was the moment I took my first baby step in the direction of the real me.

I turned the key in the ignition and pressed the gas to go. There was no turning back.

I drove out of the parking lot away from that doctor, and headed for an unknown abyss. I drove away because I had to, even though I had no idea where I was going or what was coming next. Just as well

I didn't know because I wouldn't have understood what a good and profound decision I had just made for myself about me.

I drove home, called the good doctor's office and cancelled my appointment for next year's spinal tap. The good doctor was probably excellent with lab rats but if he needed spinal fluid for his research experiments he was going to have to tap somebody else's spine. I threw away the card with the number to call for my wheelchair. I didn't see another neurologist for many years. I went somewhere else and eventually with a lot of patient help I learned who I was.

Segment 2 – Waiting for Us

As in any journey,

some people have dropped along the way,

have had enough for this round,

Others have been waiting for us to catch up.

Ram Dass
Grist for the Mill

Aura Guy

Between the time the orthopedic surgeon booked the MRI and when it was actually done, I had to talk to somebody. It couldn't be just anybody. It certainly couldn't be someone from the traditional Western medical establishment. All I had heard from them was crazy stuff. A brain tumour? A tumour on my spine? And what was this garbage about multiple sclerosis? I felt like I was being chased so doctors could slap a great big "L" on my forehead for Loser. There was no way I was going to get a fair hearing from them. I had to talk to somebody who could speak my language, who understood where I was coming from so when I said something that might sound a little *out there* I would be heard.

The first person who came to mind was a GP I had met ten years earlier. I hadn't met him in the context of a medical doctor so I was able to get to know him and enjoy his personality without the label. At the time I met him, he was studying to become a psychotherapist. I hadn't seen him in those ten years since but I had recommended him to a couple of people and they had reported he was terrific and thanked me for the lead.

I called his office and the receptionist said they had a waiting list but it was closed currently. They expected they would be reviewing it come August or September and I should phone back then. This was February; the beginning of February. I took a chance and left my name and number and also let her know that I was a friend of his. That was a bit of a stretch but it was worth a shot.

I sat there thinking for a few minutes. Who could I talk to... suddenly I remembered a card I had in my wallet. A year earlier, a friend of mine who knew everything there was to know about what was going on in Edmonton in terms of new and exciting treatments, practitioners, and general New Age info, had highly recommended a massage therapist to me. I made an appointment with this woman for a massage and my friend was right. The massage therapist was terrific. She spoke about a fellow she knew who she thought I would enjoy working with. She gave me one of his cards. I asked her what he did and she said he worked with colors. He could tell me all sorts of things about myself just by looking at my aura. When I asked her how much a session with him cost she said a hundred dollars but for that money he gave you an entire morning or afternoon of his time. It was definitely worth it she said. I didn't have any particular problems that warranted spending that kind of time and money but I really liked the card. The drawing on it was quite unique. It depicted the chakras with their different colors. That's what she told me they were. I didn't know about chakras but I really liked the drawing. I put the card in my wallet and forgot about it. That's where it had been since.

I looked through the wallet, found the card and dialed the phone number on it. There was a recording so I left a message. Fifteen minutes later Dan called back. He might as well have been speaking Chinese because I didn't understand a word he said. I must have said something but I don't remember what. When we got to the end of the conversation he said "I can work with you. Do you want to work with me?" Yes, I said and he suggested we meet Wednesday afternoon at his office because it would be quiet. He had an office in a chiropractor's clinic and the clinic closed Wednesday afternoons.

In retrospect, I broke every rule in the book for how single ladies should be careful. I went to a building I had never been to before, to an office that was in the basement, where the chiropractor's clinic would be closed, to see a man I had never met before, whose work I didn't have a clue about, with $100 in my pocket that he knew I would have, and I didn't tell anyone where I was going. Why was I so stupid? It was his voice. There was something about his voice that was reassuring and familiar. From all reports, serial killer Ted Bundy was a charming guy, too. But for some reason I totally trusted that voice and I followed it.

Friend of Aura Guy

I didn't have to explain a thing to Dan when I met him that first time. He explained more to me about me and my life than I could ever have imagined. I felt overwhelmed and validated at the same time. I was floundering in the confusion, fear and upset of what might be wrong with me physically so I was probably in a state of shock when Dan sent me home with assignments to work on after that first meeting. According to him, I needed to do a whole lot of emotional homework. There was a meditation he gave me that had to do with breathing and the colors of the chakras. I was going to have to look up what chakras were exactly. There must be a book I could get.

He told me to come back after the MRI was done so he could work on me to clean up the effect the MRI would have on my brains. I wasn't sure what he meant by that but it was fine with me if he could fix it.

Ten days later I was back in Dan's office with the confirmed diagnosis of MS. I lay on the treatment table while Dan had his hands on my head working the cranial plates. He was making adjustments to my brains to ensure they wouldn't be "fragile" following the MRI session. When he finished sorting out my MRI-scrambled brains, he called Kevin the chiropractor into his office. I only caught a glimpse of him walking past the treatment table. He pulled a chair up to the top of the table, sat down and put his hands on either side of my head. Dan introduced us. I said hello while Kevin's fingers moved around my skull. The two of them exchanged a few remarks and it turned out Kevin spoke the same, mostly incomprehensible language Dan did. After a few silent minutes concentrating on the movement of his fingers around my skull, Kevin declared that my brains were sorted, confirming the work Dan had done. He left as quickly as he arrived saying it was nice to meet me as he went out the door. I still didn't get a good look at him.

Dan explained that they had developed a language of vibration that they used to communicate with each other more precisely about what was happening with someone they were working with so they could clearly and correctly work with that person. I thought as long as the two of them understood each other, I was in and who knew? Maybe in time I would learn to recognize some of their vocabulary.

Dan suggested I start working with Kevin regularly with a trip back to his office every now and then. I got a standing appointment with Kevin for chiropractic treatments every two weeks after that and so the routine for the next two years was set.

Modality Smorgasbord

For the first two years following my diagnosis, I had a pretty good time deluding myself with how on top of things I was, how much I understood about my condition and how it was only a matter of time before I got my world back on track. I made Dan and Kevin my baseline. They were solid, ergo, so was I -- strength by association. With a starting point as strong as the two of them, I conducted my search for the right treatment, the right practice and practitioner or finding just the right vitamin that would answer my quest and end the MS. I would return to home base at the chiropractor's basement clinic for one of my regularly scheduled appointments to re-group, laugh, feel better and head out again to continue my search for answers.

I dabbled in all kinds of New Age alternative treatments and practices. I stayed in touch with the friend who had suggested I go for that wonderful massage. I could call her up and say "What's new?" and she would have an answer. I did a little foot reflexology, naturopathic drops, a lot of massage, a little acupuncture, another chiropractor here, a different chiropractor there, vitamin and mineral programs, tried meditation, Tai Chi, saltwater pools, yoga, and read the latest self-help books. I jumped from one thing to the next and I always felt better for a little while but the feeling would fade. So, I'd be back on the phone to my friend – "What's new?" And off I'd go again to explore something else.

In between phone calls to her looking for the next flavour of the month, I would go back to Dan and Kevin, Kevin and Dan, and they always welcomed me back with patience, kindness and a smile. I would have great sessions with them and then off I'd go on another modality adventure.

For two years I lived in that fantasy land, acting like I understood it all and everything was going to be fine. I was still walking sort of okay as long as it was fewer than six city blocks round-trip. I could still drive but I only went around town on well-known favourite routes outside of rush-hour traffic and I didn't go on the highway. Overall, if I wasn't operating at one hundred per cent then I was operating at a solid sixty-five per cent.

There was always some new, hot, trendy, modality to check out but for all the new treatments and practices I tried, the place that was consistent, the one I went back to again and again was the basement clinic on 82nd Avenue with Kevin the chiropractor and Dan with the Pied Piper's voice. They were fascinating people and I always felt better being there. They gave me lots of *you-can-do-it* attitude, which I soaked up like a dry sponge that's been left out in the rain.

Coming Apart at the Sacrum

One day in March, 1997 that friend who had her finger on the pulse of Edmonton's New Age community invited me to go with her to a morning of meditation with a group she had discovered recently. *Oh good*, I thought, *a group meditation. I will think my way out of the multiple sclerosis using the added energy of a group vibration.* My friend spoke particularly well about the woman who conducted the meditation sessions from her home. I accepted her invitation and on a bright, sunny, winter morning she drove us to this woman's acreage outside the city.

The Thursday morning meditation group had half a dozen students. As it turned out, I wasn't as happy with the session as I hoped I would be. In fact, I was flat out bored but I hung in there and participated as best I could. The other people attending seemed to be very keen about it all.

On the drive back to Edmonton I wasn't comfortable. It felt like my lower back was becoming unhinged. That's the best way to describe what I felt. It wasn't painful but it felt like my lower back was coming apart one vertebra after the other. By the time I got home, walking was much more difficult than usual.

I had left my job at the real estate development company the year before and was working three days a week at the Red Cross office on the south side of Edmonton. I had to go to work the next day. I asked my father to drive me to and from the office because I knew I couldn't. My lower back was not connecting well with my legs. On the weekend, my father went to a medical supply store and purchased a cane to help me get around. By Tuesday, when my father drove me to my late afternoon appointment at the clinic with Kevin, I was completely dependent on that cane. In the space of one morning my body had turned on me. The diagnosis of MS was a betrayal on paper that I had blithely treated with this modality or another but this sudden new development was a physical betrayal that was horribly real and frightening.

Finally, They Had My Attention

I sat in the clinic's waiting area with three other patients who were leafing through magazines. It was late afternoon and the receptionist had already gone home for the day. I was sitting in a chair beside the wall with the cane on the floor hidden between the wall and the chair legs. Dan came out of his office dressed in his coat and hat, his backpack slung over his shoulder. He was on his way home. It was March and it had been snowing most of the day.

When Dan saw me, he stopped at the corner of the empty reception desk. He looked at me and said hi. The other three waiting patients immediately looked up. I said hi back. He cocked his head a little to one side and said "How are you?" I knew better than to lie and say fine. He was looking at me in that way I had become familiar with where I knew *he* knew, so I said, "I've been better." He didn't say anything. He just walked away. The door to the clinic closed behind him. I heard his boots clomping up the staircase and then he was gone.

Dan? I was surprised and disappointed that he didn't say anything else. I thought maybe he didn't really see what was happening with me. I wanted to tell him all about it and what a lousy weekend I had lived through but I didn't want to say anything personally significant in front of all these strangers who were suddenly perky and interested in what the two of us might have to say.

I waited for my turn to see Kevin while the other three people had their appointments before me. Finally, it was my turn. I was the last one. Kevin opened the door to his office and said "Hi, Cath. Come on in." I reached for the cane on the floor and stood up. I took a very unsteady step and waited a moment to get my balance. I looked up to see just how far I had to go to get to his office door but what I saw was Kevin's stony face. Two years I had been coming to the clinic and I had never seen him look that way before.

He didn't move. He didn't try to help me. He just stood there as I made my way one wobbly step after the other. When I finally got to the office door, he stepped aside and took my arm closing the door behind me. He helped me over to the treatment table and sat me down on it. He asked me what had happened and all I could say was I didn't know, that it started a couple of days ago.

He went to the phone and dialed a number. I knew he was trying to call Dan so I told him I didn't know where Dan lived but he wouldn't be home yet. It was snowing outside and the traffic was moving slowly. When there was no answer he hung up the phone and started to do the session with me. A little while later he went back to the phone and tried calling Dan again. This time there was an answer and Kevin left a message to have Dan call the office as soon as he got in. Kevin asked me if I could stick around until Dan phoned back but I couldn't. My father had brought me to the appointment and he was upstairs waiting in the car. If I kept him waiting any longer it wouldn't go over very well. After all, he had done me a great favour by taking me to and from work and now he was sitting in his car waiting for me at my chiropractor's appointment. The driving conditions were deteriorating and it was really close to dinner time. I had exhausted my allotment of favours from him for the week.

Kevin got me to the bottom of the staircase just as my father appeared at the top. He was wondering where I was and how much longer I was going to be. Kevin called him "sir" and spoke to him respectfully. It was as if he'd read the tension in my father's attitude and did his best to defuse the man's hostility. I managed to get up the stairs and we went home.

The Observer Breakthrough

Three days later my father drove me home from work again. It was Friday. He walked me up the stairs to my third floor apartment one step at a time. How I wished my wonderful apartment building had an elevator. When I got into my apartment I sat down on the couch exhausted. My father asked me if I was going to be okay and I said yes. He left for home. I sat on the couch trying to figure out what I was going to make for dinner after my legs had recovered from climbing the stairs. Whatever I made, it was going to have to be simple. I couldn't stand longer than the time it took to make a sandwich.

I hadn't heard from Kevin or Dan since my appointment three days earlier. The voice in my head started its usual negative yammering. *Maybe they don't want to see you again. Two years of being there for you and you show up with a cane. Ingrate. Who could blame them if they showed you the door? "Here's your cane, Loser. Don't let the door hit you on the way out."*

It was silent in my apartment. I didn't have the strength to walk across the room, pick up the remote control and turn on the television. The stereo was in the same area as the TV so I couldn't get to that either. I sat there thinking in the quiet but it wasn't about what to make for dinner. I was wondering how I got into this state. I could barely walk. *How did that happen? What did I do?*

The phone rang. It was Dan.

He said he couldn't figure it out like he'd been listening to my thoughts. Kevin didn't know what was going on either. They thought – I stopped him in midsentence. "I know when it started,' I said. The words were out of my mouth before I realized what I was going to say. It was spontaneous interruption without forethought.

"When?" he asked.

"I was in the car coming home from the morning meditation session when it felt like my lower back was coming apart."

"What morning meditation session?" he wanted to know. I didn't usually tell Dan and Kevin about my forays into the latest New Age modality adventure until after the fact. I thought of those exploits as separate activities unrelated to my appointments with them.

"The one I was invited to go to," I answered.

"Who invited you?" he prompted. I gave him the name of my friend who had driven me out there and back.

"Out where?" was his next question. I told him we had gone to an acreage owned by the lady who did this weekly meditation group my friend had been going to.

"Who's the lady?" he asked. When I said her name, he practically came through the phone at me. Apparently my answer had caught him off guard but he knew who I was talking about and suddenly it all made sense to him. I put the phone back to my ear. He apologized immediately. Now it was my turn for questions.

"Who is she?" I asked. No, he couldn't tell me.

"Why not?" I persisted. Because he had had a run-in with her some years back and he didn't want his personal opinion about her to influence what my experience of her might have been.

"Dan," I said, "I'm sitting on the couch and I can't raise one leg to cross it over the other. Tell me."

There was silence for a moment while he thought about it and then he let loose with the story. His unedited opinions were generously peppered with colorful adjectives. I had never heard him speak so openly or frankly about something he felt that strongly about. When he took a breath, I asked him if this woman's meditation session could have affected me so that I reacted with my spine becoming unhinged. I listened to his explanation and while I didn't understand most of it, what I heard was it probably did have that impact on me.

It seemed like we were on the phone for a long time and in the end he was relieved. He was relieved because it wasn't something he had said that set me off and put me in the state I was in. He was relieved it wasn't anything Kevin had done. He kept saying "Wait 'til Kevin hears this." Now that he had the context for why my condition had shifted so quickly, they could work with it.

I felt better, too. Dan was talking to me like I was a friend, and we had a shared experience, like I was someone he could trust. I felt special that he had confided in me, albeit loudly. They weren't mad at me. There could be a real reason why my health had taken such a scary turn so fast. Maybe it wasn't my body going wacko against me in a senseless MS attack. Maybe they could fix it. Maybe I should tell them next time where I'm going *before* I go just in case it could have unwanted repercussions. Maybe I should stick with them and quit running around all over the place on my modality adventures.

After I got off the phone with Dan, I realized I had never taken the time to sit quietly and think about what I had been doing prior to something different occurring. I don't know why I started to think like that on this day. In my normal able-bodied brain, the way I did things was to keep charging ahead, on to the next thing. I didn't stop and think – what just happened here? But, for some reason, I did this time – when I didn't have the strength to get up off the couch, cross the room to get the remote control and distract myself with TV. Instead, I sat in the silence and asked myself, *when did this start happening?* When I remembered being in the car and remembered the feeling of my tailbone coming undone, I did something I had never done before. I made a connection between my present circumstance and what I had been thinking, feeling and doing just before my present circumstance occurred. Maybe two years of sessions at the clinic with Kevin and Dan had made an impression on me. Maybe what they had been trying to teach me had started to sink in. *Miracle of miracles. The power of observation – cause and effect.*

I sat in silence and connected the dots. My view of the world – and me in it – had dislodged.

"If You Think I was a Mess, You Should Have Seen Him"

<hr>

"Wait till Kevin hears this." Dan said that since I'd made my stumbling appearance in their office three days earlier, he and Kevin had been yelling at each other. Dan thought Kevin had done something and Kevin thought Dan had said something to set me off and put me on a cane. He was so relieved my crumbling condition had nothing to do with the work they had done with me that he could hardly contain himself. Dan knew the woman who conducted the morning meditation session and in his experience with her, she had apparently tripped some issue in me that was the cause for my back "unhooking." He was talking so fast I didn't really get it all but that was okay. He did, and to me that meant this was fixable. I had identified the circumstance and he understood it.

Then Dan said, "If you think I was a mess, you should have seen him."

Excuse me?

Dan said when he saw me in the clinic waiting area that day he was so stunned by how I appeared to him that he couldn't believe what he was seeing. From the way he looks at the world, what he saw when he looked at me he described as "road kill." He said by the time he got to the top of the stairs after leaving the office to go outside he was crying. He didn't go home. He said he walked around the block for an hour, crying, thinking, trying to figure out what had happened to me. When he got back to the office I was gone and he found Kevin in much the same state he was. He said they had been yelling at each other ever since trying to figure out how I got so messed up.

Hearing Dan's description of how he and Kevin had reacted to seeing me on a cane amazed me. Dan had cried? Kevin had cried? They had been yelling at each other, accusing each other of being responsible for causing this unexpected health reversal? I don't remember ever having heard or seen a man upset for me, let alone two. Their reaction to seeing me on a cane shocked me. We shocked each other that day, I guess.

I had my next appointment with Kevin on the following Tuesday afternoon. He helped me onto the treatment table. When I was lying there, he picked up my right hand. He held my hand in one of his and caressed it with the other. He wasn't looking at me. He was looking at my hand. After a moment he said, "I don't think you realize what you mean to Dan and me."

What?

If I hadn't already been lying down I would've fallen down. I meant something to the two of them? I was floored. I had never experienced tenderness like that from a man and it made me very uncomfortable. Where I came from, a man showing tenderness was a sign of weakness. To be sentimental and sweet and gentle was to be mocked, put down and made fun of. I reacted by doing what I knew how to do which was say something stupid, which I did. I don't remember exactly what I said and that's probably a good thing. I just remember after I said it, Kevin looked at me and smiled. He put my hand down and we had our session.

Kevin was right. I didn't know what I meant to them. For two years, they had taken my situation seriously and invested their time, energy, knowledge and experience in my case. They were genuinely interested in their work and wanted to help people live better lives. They had gotten to know me and wanted to know how I was doing. They wanted to know how their efforts were working for me. For two years, I flounced around playing *Name That Modality*. I hadn't considered that I was doing as well as I was because of their awareness and plain hard work. And, it turns out, they liked me just like I liked them.

After two years, the Universe had my attention and Dan and Kevin finally had a real live student to work with.

The Guardian Angel of Gimps

The chiropractor's office was in the basement of an historic building in Old Strathcona. Old Strathcona is an older section of Edmonton that has evolved from the original city site on the south side of the North Saskatchewan River to a popular trendy neighborhood. The area is represented primarily by one street – Whyte – also known as 82nd Avenue. Restaurants, bars and funky shops line both sides of the road. Not only is Old Strathcona popular with Edmontonians, it's also the site of one of the city's major summer festivals, the Fringe Festival. Other than that, 82nd Avenue is the straight line east-west corridor to the University of Alberta and the University of Alberta Hospital. It's a busy street.

Needless to say, parking in front of the building that the chiropractor's office was in was a challenge. There were meters on both sides of the street but I thought getting one of those spots was virtually impossible. There was a big open lot about five blocks away that I would park in but five blocks was a long way for me to walk and after I got to the building I had to walk down a flight of stairs to the office in the basement. I really had to get one of those meter spaces on 82nd Avenue as close to the building as I could possibly get. I just did not have the leg strength for a five-block walk and a flight of stairs.

I would cruise the block again and again looking for an empty space telling the cars to move and grumbling about their selfish owners who were nowhere to be seen. How did people get these spaces? How come I couldn't get one? I needed one. These people were shopping or eating or generally wasting my time and my energy. Around and around I went, complaining about these nameless, self-interested people whose only purpose in life seemed to be to frustrate the daylights out of me. When I wasn't completely consumed with grumbling, every now and then I would have some success. The meter I got might be at the end of the block but never mind. It was better than walking five.

One day before I left for my appointment, I got into my car in the underground garage of the condo I had moved to and just sat there. I started praying. *Please, please, please I have to have a parking space on 82nd right in front of the building, right in front of the door. I don't have the energy to walk a block today. I have to get to that appointment. It will make me feel better. Please, please, please I need that parking space right in front of the door.* I pictured the spot in my mind. I knew where I had to be. *Please, please, please.* I started the engine and drove out of the garage. I prayed all the way there. Driving down the street, stopping at a red light, driving across the High Level Bridge, turning onto Saskatchewan Dr., turning south on 104th Street and stopping at the red light at 104th and 82nd Avenue, I sat there praying. *Please, please, please, when the light changes and I turn on to 82nd please, please, please let there be a parking space right in front of the door.* The light changed. I turned the corner and crept by every parked car on the south side of the street. *Please, please, please.* And then just ahead I saw a car pull out from the meters in front of me. I was going slowly so the driver had time to pull out in front of me and get into the flow of traffic.

He pulled out of the space I wanted right in front of the door of the building my chiropractor's office was in.

I pulled into the spot before anyone else had a chance to see it. I turned off the engine and sat there amazed and thrilled. My prayers changed from please, please, please, to thank you, thank you, thank you. I got out of the car, walked around to the meter and plugged it with all the quarters I needed to save the spot for two hours. I walked across the sidewalk up the step and opened the front door of the building. I walked across the black-and-white tiled lobby and down the stairs to the chiropractor's office. I was so excited I told everybody I talked to that I had the metered parking space in front of the building. I was laughing and talking about it and somewhere along the line the words 'guardian angel' came up. From that day on I prayed to the Guardian Angel of Gimps for my metered parking space in front of the building my chiropractor's office was in and from that day on I always got it. It never failed. I would think about the parking space before I left home and picture it in my mind and I would ask the Guardian Angel of Gimps to please save that spot for me. The space was always available when I drove up.

I always thought of the angel as female. I don't know why. But she never let me down. At the chiropractor's office the parking space in front of the building became known as my space.

On a few occasions there was another car parked in my space but the meter behind it was available. I would park in the available space and keep the engine running. I would sit there blessing the person who owned the car that was parked in my space instead of grumbling about him or her. I would bless them with having a great day and getting all their shopping done quickly and efficiently and finding everything they needed. I would explain that I needed the space they were parked in because I had a chiropractor's appointment and my legs were weak. I would bless them some more saying I knew they understood and wanted to be helpful. I just kept up chatter like that in my head all the while blessing the car owner with the very best things I could think of. Usually, it only took a couple of minutes but by golly the owner of the car would show up, get in the car and drive off. When the car drove off I drove forward and slipped into the vacated parking space. Pretty soon, not only was that spot available for me whenever I requested it but when I went to put coins in the meter, I would discover there was still time on it from the previous occupant.

That was the first tangible evidence I had that if I knew what I wanted, could picture it clearly in my mind, and ask for it with some emotion behind the request, I would get it. I would get what I asked for or something better. I always remembered to say thank you.

I began to think something out there was listening. I was raised Catholic so thinking about a guardian angel was a familiar concept for me. It was like a person but invisible with magic powers. It was handy to have a connection to a being like that. I hadn't thought about guardian angels since grade school and it was nice to remember that I had one especially when it got me the perfect parking space. I started to experiment with other things I needed like a new winter coat for the price I had budgeted. My requests were always answered and it usually didn't take very long to get positive answers either.

I always put my requests out there for some other kind of magic being to handle for me. I never thought that it was me being the one who was creating the magic. And all of my requests were something I needed, something I could justify having. I never asked for something that could be considered fun or frivolous or maybe something I wanted, simply wanted. I could justify a request for something I needed but asking for something I wanted was self-indulgent. Other people got what they wanted. Not me.

When I started telling people about the Guardian Angel of Gimps and my perfect parking space, I found out a lot of them could also manifest parking spaces for themselves. They weren't gimps or Catholic and they didn't use a guardian angel but they were just as successful getting great parking spots anywhere they wanted.

Imagining a Guardian Angel of Gimps put me back into a space that had a spiritual framework that had been missing from my life for a long time. I didn't realize it then though. Requesting parking spaces was still under the heading of some kind of game I played, but it did get results I couldn't ignore. I began to realize that identifying what it was I needed could also be something I wanted. If I identified it clearly and asked, I could trust that there would be a response. I could trust my request. I would be heard.

Segment 3 – Lose Sight of Land

One doesn't discover new lands

without consenting

to lose sight of the shore

for a very long time.

Andre Gide

Treading Water

I was terrified but I was trying to hang onto my life with everything I had. I was losing my health just as the doctors had predicted. I felt lousy. I had no energy. Whatever strength I had was going, going, gone and the fatigue was crippling -- no pun intended. I couldn't keep up with my job anymore. The two fellows I worked for had tried all kinds of arrangements so that I could keep working but no matter what we tried to do I came up lacking. No matter how hard I tried I couldn't work a five day week anymore the way I used to, the way I wanted to. When there were no more options left, I did. It was May, 1996.

I took some time off, rested up and then got myself a temporary job at the Red Cross blood donor office in a secretarial position. It was five days a week again but the pace was a bit slower than the development company and I lucked out meeting a group of women who worked there. They kept me laughing all day long. But that five days a week routine got to me again. Fortunately, the Red Cross office also had part-time positions available. If I really wasn't up to working five days a week as I had just proved to myself again, then

I would work three. I could still see my new friends at lunch every other day. They kept me laughing even when I had to start using a cane. Maybe I should say they kept me laughing, especially when they saw me with the cane.

Following another uproarious lunch, a woman who worked in the office also on a temporary basis, commented to me with a scowl that she didn't know how I could take all those remarks. I told her I would crawl to work to hear those hysterical lines from those fabulous ladies. She didn't hear the kindness or the concern or the friendship in their voices and I didn't explain it.

Every day, I pretended that everything was fine, but really it wasn't. On the outside, everything looked great at work but inside I was afraid and angry. The fear was new. The anger wasn't. I was mad at the world, I was mad at God and I let Him know it with both barrels on a regular basis. I hung onto Dan and Kevin like they were tree trunks being swept down the same river I was being swallowed by at spring thaw. They were afloat and kept my head above water as long as I was holding on to them. Their clinic was the safe place.

I moved from my third-floor apartment to an apartment on the second floor. I had lived on the third floor of that building for four-teen years but now I had to move because I couldn't climb that many stairs anymore. My parents and friends helped me move. I consoled myself with the fact that I didn't have to leave the building. I loved the location – just up the hill from the North Saskatchewan River where the geese gathered in the fall before they headed south and deer came by the parking lot in winter to chew on bare tree branches. I was glad I didn't have to leave.

So I was okay. I had lost some of my health but I could get that back. I had found Dan and Kevin and they believed I could get better. I had lost my job at the real estate development company but the two fellows I worked for and their families were still friends, so that was great. I was working, albeit part-time. That meant my income wasn't so terrific but I had made wonderful new friends. I was still living in the same building so being one floor down from where I had been was no big deal. I made a few adjustments, added a cane to my wardrobe and carried on like it was all just fine.

The Pronouncement

My parents liked the area I lived in so when they moved to Edmonton in 1988 they asked if I would mind if they moved into my neighbourhood. That was fine with me. They lived on the same street a couple of blocks away and that proved to be handy now when I needed help following my diagnosis. They were wonderful, helping me with chores as I found it increasingly difficult to do food shopping, for example. I was trying really hard to do my best to keep my life together at the same time as it was slipping out of my hands. Dwindling strength and sometimes overwhelming fatigue were making my life an hourly struggle.

One Saturday afternoon in the early summer of 1997, my father arrived at my apartment to tell me that all this going back and forth between our apartments trying to live their lives and helping me with mine was "crap" and it had to stop. I was told that he and my mother had been going out whenever they had a free minute looking at apartments that we could move into together. I was told that after an extensive search they had found the one and only three-bedroom apartment that existed in the city of Edmonton. I was told they had spoken to the building manager and explained our situation and the manager was willing to hold the apartment until I had had a chance to see it. I was told we had to make a decision quickly because the one and only three-bedroom apartment in all of Edmonton would be rented quickly. Even though all these arrangements had been made by my parents and it was obviously a done deal, I still asked if I could have a day to think about it. My father said I had until tomorrow and he left.

I knew what he really wanted was for me to say terrific, let's go right now. I know that's what he had in mind and it was pretty brazen of me to ask if I could have a day to think about it, but if I had asked if I could have time without stipulating how much, that would've been completely unacceptable. My father would likely have gone ballistic and made me feel like I was the scum of the earth. So I asked for a day.

What I really needed was air. I was so shocked by his declaration, breathing had become an afterthought. I was stunned that my parents had made this decision that we should move to a new place and live together without including me in the conversation. I was stunned that as often as we saw and spoke to each other, they had done all this decision-making and running around behind my back. They had never said a word about what they were thinking or doing or what their intentions were. I was stunned that they felt it was perfectly acceptable for my father to arrive unannounced and drop this bombshell in my lap without so much as a hello-goodbye. I was stunned that my parents felt they could unilaterally and so dramatically pull the rug right out from underneath me without including me in the discussion. I was forty-four years old, not three. I had this rotten miserable disease and I was trying so hard. They might as well have each taken a turn and slapped me across the face.

If I had said, "Hey, wait a minute!", or God forbid, "no", my parents would have likely taken the position that it was their way or the highway. If I didn't get on board with their plan, the implied threat was they would cut me off and abandon me. As a youngster, this was a highly effective strategy with me. And now I was reacting as a child again. I was so afraid to be left behind without help that I shut up and went along with what was expected. They were being generous, wanting to help and figuring out how we could do it. It was my job to be grateful and compliant.

My father's visit that Saturday afternoon made the reality of my situation brilliantly clear in an instant. I had lost my health, I had lost my job and now I was being handed a doubleheader – I was going to lose the place I had called home for more than fourteen years and whatever fantasies I had about being independent, self-sufficient and coping with a physical challenge.

We went to see the one and only three-bedroom apartment in all of Edmonton the next day.

The Homeowner's Detour

The apartment door opened into a large room with big windows that faced west. It was bright and sunny and looked like there would be a lot of space but the room was supposed to be both the living and dining rooms. There was a kitchen that was a pretty good size that opened onto the large room but there was no dishwasher. There was only one bathroom and three "bedrooms". The "master bedroom" was about the size of an average kid's room and the other two bedrooms were walk-in closets. My parents worked very hard to get me as enthusiastic about the apartment as they were. They suggested I could have the master bedroom and they would take one of the other bedrooms. I could set up the third bedroom as my own TV room. They had a queen size bed and a beautiful rock maple bureau. There was no way they could have gotten both of those pieces of furniture in one of the other bedrooms never mind with the two end tables on either side of the bed. They would have had to put the bed in one bedroom, the bureau in the other and sell the end tables.

I was trying really hard not to cry. When I was asked if we should take the apartment I said no. Big mistake. One did not say no to my father without his anger being made very clear. Afterwards, I sat in the front seat of the car beside him on the way to the grocery store where my mother had to pick up a couple of items for dinner. He was so angry the atmosphere in the car was suffocating. I decided then and there that the very next apartment we saw I would say yes to no matter what it was and put us all out of our misery.

When we got to the grocery store I suggested they might pick up one of those renters guides so we could look through and see what else might be available in Edmonton. On the back of the guide they picked up was a full page ad for an apartment complex in the west end of the city. It read beautifully. When we got back home my father called the number. Yes, they had a three-bedroom apartment available. We got back in the car immediately and drove straight to that complex to check it out. Apparently there was more than one three-bedroom apartment in Edmonton.

The apartment we were shown was much larger than the one we had seen earlier and it was much better divided. All the rooms were a decent size and there were two full bathrooms. The second bathroom was an en suite with the master bedroom adjacent to a walk-in closet. My parents were happy and when they asked me if I could live in that apartment I said yes. My father was thrilled and life with him became bearable again.

Wonderful friends again helped me to pack up my apartment. I gave away a lot of what I had but I couldn't give it all away or sell it. I ended up with my favourite framed pictures and thirteen boxes of what I considered to be precious, important, and necessary items for when I got my next place and could set up a new home for myself. My former boss stored those thirteen boxes and framed pictures in his basement after his wife and kids collected them from me. Little did I know and little did they know that those boxes and pictures would stay in their basement for the next seven years.

We stayed in the west end apartment for almost a year. It was in one of the low-rise apartment buildings in the complex. The project was always busy with people coming and going. There was also one high-rise apartment building. When the front of one of the prefab concrete balconies on the high-rise fell to the ground from the seventh floor, my father decided it was time to go. We broke our lease, which cost us some money, and went looking for another place to live.

My father was determined to find a house but none of the houses we saw in our price range piqued our interest. My mother and I finally managed to convince my father that we should look at a condo and not a house by pointing out the fact that if we had a house we would be required to shovel snow-covered sidewalks and mow our lawn -- neither of which he had any interest in doing any more. We weren't having much success with our search. Then my parents asked me if the bank could assess what I was worth and we could add that to the kitty. I was thrilled. This was not only acknowledgment that I existed but if the bank thought I was worth something financially, I could make a contribution to this effort. On paper I wasn't worth all that much but I felt great to be part of the game plan.

Shortly afterward we found a condo that worked for us. It was a cozy fit but it had a few features that were excellent for three adults living together. The two bedrooms were on either side of the apartment. There were two full bathrooms and one of those bathrooms was en suite as in a master bedroom, which I occupied. There was a separate sunroom that was large enough for my father and I to divide into two offices – one for him and one for me. The sunroom could be closed off from the rest of the apartment with sliding glass doors. We signed the deal and my name was included as one of the owners. I had never owned any kind of real estate before. It had never occurred to me that I could own real estate on my own so I had never investigated the possibility. What a wasted opportunity. I liked being an owner.

Tangled Expectations

We lived in that condo for seven years. I loved the neighborhood. It was north of the river on the west side of the downtown area. In the spring of that year a friend of mine offered me a job working as a contributing writer for the marketing department he worked in. I could work at home and go to the office for meetings or when they needed to see the whites of my eyes. The office was six blocks away from the condo we bought. Best of all, Earl's Restaurant, with the most popular patio in the city, was at the end of my street a half block away. I got to know a couple of the hostesses there so that I didn't have to make a reservation. I could show up on my scooter, say how many people I was meeting, and get a table. Considering how popular the patio was on a sunny Friday afternoon, having that kind of access was saying a lot. So, some aspects of my new reality were working.

Forty-four and Living
with Mum and Dad

Three adults living in the same space, two of those adults are a long-time married couple and the parents of the third adult, their child whose physical disability is gradually worsening. This is a formula for tension.

I left home at 19. I had a roommate, a friend I had made during first year university. Apart from that, I had pretty much lived on my own since. I had lived in various apartments in Calgary, moved to Banff twice for short-term jobs, back to Calgary and then moved to Edmonton over the space of twenty-five years. I had pretty much figured out my likes and dislikes, and what I did like was living on my own and having my independence. Suddenly, I was trying to cope with a body that wasn't working right, needing help, losing my independence, and moving back in with Mum and Dad. Those were shocks to my psyche on every count.

Fortunately, the layout of the condo we moved into was good. It had two bedrooms each with its own bathroom. One bedroom and bathroom were on either side of the condo separated by the kitchen, dining room and living room. My parents generously suggested I take the master bedroom with its en suite bathroom while they took the second bedroom. There was also a wonderful sunroom that ran the length of my bedroom and the width of the living room. There were big glass windows in the sunroom so even though we faced north that room was always light compared to the rest of the apartment.

The sunroom was large enough that we were able to divide it in half by using a bookshelf my parents had. On one side of the bookshelf my father had his office set up with his computer and on the other side of the bookshelf I had my office with computer, love seat and television. There was an entrance from the master bedroom to my side of the sunroom and there were glass sliding doors from the living room to my father's side of the sunroom. At night, when my parents were watching television in the living room, they could close the glass sliding doors so neither of us was disturbed by watching conflicting programs on either of our television sets. During the day, I worked in my half of the sunroom while my father was away at the office. It was a good workspace. On weekends, my parents would leave the condo as many as three times a day doing the food shopping, going on other errands or just going for a drive to see what was new around town and getting a coffee somewhere. That was their way of giving each of us our own space. Sometimes when I knew they were going out for a drive and a coffee that made me so sad because I couldn't get out and around as easily as they could – as easily as I used to be able to do.

My parents wanted to help me. I expected them to help me. They felt the responsibility and the obligation to help their physically challenged adult child. The problem as far as I was concerned was that the help they offered was not the way I wanted to be helped. I tried with every ounce of strength and angry determination I had to prove that I could cope, that nothing really had changed that much, that I could still live my own life. I had my way of doing things and how I wanted them done.

Unfortunately, at the time, my version of multiple sclerosis was a fluid condition. If my condition had been the same every day, then my parents and I could have stood on some kind of stable footing – all puns intended. We could have adjusted or compromised our way of doing things and established a consistent routine but my MS symptoms moved, shifted and changed sometimes on an hourly basis. One moment I was bright and felt well and the next moment I had the strength of an overcooked noodle with a foggy brain to match. All three of us were trying to cope but we never knew what the next hour would be like, never mind the next day.

My parents wanted to help me and I needed their help but I wanted them to help me *my* way. They wanted to do things for me *their* way. I wanted to try. They were uncomfortable watching me try especially when I wasn't successful on the first few attempts. They wanted to do *for* me. That led to a lot of misunderstandings, frustration and flat out anger from each of us. I was told that I should just tell them what it was I wanted and on those rare occasions when I did get up the nerve to say what it was I really wanted, I would be made to feel like I had just ruined their day. That attitude was particularly true from my father. I was made to feel that I had asked for the impossible, and they resented my request. I was told on more than one occasion how their efforts to help me were continually met by my anger and they were fed up with being made to feel that their attempts to help were miserable failures. It was a tough situation.

When my parents and I moved in together, they were Mum and Dad and I was the child I thought they expected me to be. That's the way I reacted most of the time. I wasn't an adult, disabled or otherwise. I was the child and whether I was using a cane, supported by walking poles, or in a wheelchair, I was the crippled child. It was as if I hadn't grown up at all. When we were in each other's company, we were set in our roles as parent and child automatically, instinctively, and by force of habit.

Babe Meets The Ugly Duckling

Babe was a pig who could herd sheep because he had been raised by border collies. The Ugly Duckling wasn't ugly or a duckling. He was a swan who broke through his egg shell into the world in the wrong nest.

Three years of living with my parents and that was the silent rant I got into in the wee small hours one morning in the confines of my own head. It was dark outside except for streetlights and it was dark inside the sunroom except for the light coming from my computer. The only sound was the clicking of the computer keys as I typed. My fingers were feeling the effects of the MS and didn't type very well anymore so to sit there typing out a rant was a lot of work.

I woke up in the wee small hours quite often. If I was upset about something I would cry. If I was going to cry, I tried to keep that happening between midnight and 6 a.m. and get it out of my system before I emerged from my bedroom to eat breakfast. If I was ticked off about something I would head for my computer in the pre-dawn darkness to type out how confused, hurt, angry and alienated I felt. My parents never said if they heard me crying or typing at that hour.

This night's Babe/Ugly Duckling theme centered on the idea that somewhere along the line I figured I must have been switched at birth or perhaps adopted. I had concluded that I was definitely not in the right family. I was much too different from the people posing as my parents.

As often as my parents encouraged me to tell them what it was I wanted or needed, I usually saw those requests received like unwelcome impositions. There were certain things that were okay to ask for, like items I wanted to add to the grocery list but that didn't always work out. I was starting to have trouble with incontinence and there was a product I had seen advertised that I wanted to try. I gave my parents the name of the product and the extra money to buy it above and beyond what I usually gave them for my share of the groceries. They could get the product at the drugstore in the same strip mall the grocery store was in. When they came home from grocery shopping they didn't have the product. When I asked about it they said they would get it the next day. My mother said, "You didn't need it today, did you?" It was an incontinent product. Would they not think this was something I needed *now*? Maybe they thought if they bought it that day I would let it collect dust in the closet until whenever. A friend happened to come by that afternoon to take me out for coffee. I sat in the coffee shop and cried. When we were finished our coffees and I had stopped sniveling, we went to a drugstore and bought the product I needed.

In time, I came to believe that not only were my requests unwelcome impositions but so was I. They were my parents, I wasn't well, they wanted to help, but for me they weren't helping the right way and for them I wasn't accepting their help correctly. I was convinced I was in the wrong place. And so it was on this midnight ramble at the computer that I created the *Mallard Scenario* illustrating precisely how different and out of place I was living with my parents.

I took my brilliant conclusions to my next session with Kevin. He listened attentively as I carefully and precisely laid out my fabulous scenario. He waited patiently for me to finish my diatribe and then he smashed my outline to pieces when he gently pointed out the major flaw in my premise. Mallard or not, half of my DNA was from my mother and the other half of my DNA was from my father. Not only were my conclusions wrong but, in fact, I was exactly where I was supposed to be.

I'm supposed to be there?

After he succinctly trashed my theory and completely destroyed at least two hours of self-righteous rant done in the silent darkness before my clock radio went off, I realized I had to re-work my hypothesis.

Damn.

When the appointment was over, Kevin cheerfully carried me up the stairs to my car. When I was about to turn the key in the ignition, it hit me.

He carried me up the stairs.

He'd done it before, more than once. Sometimes he carried me down the stairs, too. He carried me in his arms like the damsel in distress. When my legs weren't having a good day my chiropractor carried me down to and up from appointments in his basement office. Why did he do that?

Because he was a nice guy and I had MS.

Because after a few years and all those appointments we were friends and I needed help. Because he was kind and had children of his own and I was a child in trouble.

Wasn't it interesting that I railed against my parents for being parents but I didn't see myself as a child when that was exactly what I was? What was wrong with this picture or rather what was skewed with my view of it?

Wow...

After much more thought about what Kevin had said, I also thought about how I had spent the bulk of my life trying to please my parents so I could win their approval. My mother's approval was easier to get than my father's. His approval was virtually non--existent and if you did win points with him for something, the points would always be tempered with a "but." Nothing was ever quite right. It would have been better if I just missed the mark. No matter how hard I tried, nothing I ever did quite met his standards.

I realized my MS was working for me in that it gave me the justification to be the child. I needed help like a child does – I literally needed to be picked up and carried. If I wanted something and I didn't get it I could blame somebody else and most of the time my parents were my easy targets. It was their fault, not mine. I couldn't help it. I had MS.

And then another understanding hit me sitting in my car. Dan had talked about being trapped in a box. I had built a box with my beliefs that allowed my MS to exist. If I broke the box down would the MS go away? If I broke the box down would I have to stop being a child? If I broke that box down would I have to be an adult? A little kid couldn't break down that box and get out of it but a grown-up could.

Did I want to get out of the box or was I comfy where I was?

God's Consolation Prize

Getting in and out of the shower was tricky and some days it worked better than others. I had grab bars put into the bathtub so I could hang onto something while I stepped into the tub, take a couple of steps to where the shower head was and hang on while I washed. My legs were feeling weaker and so were my arms, which made shampooing my medium length hair a challenge. My hair was straight and I used to use big fat Velcro rollers to make my hair look as though it had some kind of lift and body. I also owned a hair dryer, a curling iron and steam curlers. I rarely used 'product' and I never used hairspray. But holding a wire brush in one hand and a hair dryer in the other really got to be difficult.

One day while I was struggling with my hair after a shower I thought I noticed a bit of a wave on the left side of my head beside my face. Hm... odd... I noticed it again after another shower but combing my hair into place combed it away.

A couple of more hair washes went by and one day I simply combed my hair into the shape I wanted with a part and let it dry on its own. My mother came by and said --

"What did you do to your hair?"

I looked up. "What?"

"Did you curl your hair?" She wanted to know.

"No. Why?" I asked.

"You've got a ringlet," she said. "Right there."

I looked in the mirror and she was right. I had a perfectly formed ringlet framing the left side of my face. The rest of my hair was straight but there was this Shirley-Temple-wanna-be-ringlet dangling all by itself.

Over the course of the next few weeks the rest of my hair got wavier and waiver. At a session with Kevin I told him my hair was getting wavy. The news didn't seem to make much of an impression. On my next appointment I brought a picture my father had taken of me in the hallway of our condo. It showed me smiling and my shoulder length brown hair with a little bit of a turn at the bottom. I purposely did nothing with my hair following my shower that morning except give it a part and let it dry on its own

I went into Kevin's office and handed him the picture. He looked at it and didn't look up.

"That's me last summer just before my brother's wedding," I said. "And this is what I look like this morning after my shower."

Kevin looked up at me and then looked back down at the picture. He left the office saying "Has Dan seen this?"

Kevin and Dan looked at the picture, looked at me, and discussed it in their usual Dan-Kevin-speak language. Neither one was sure exactly what was happening but something obviously was. This was very exciting for me. I had tangible evidence on the top of my head that something *good* was happening for a change. I chalked it up to the work I was doing with the two of them. To me it looked like something positive had finally registered with me and wavy hair was the tangible indicator that I was on the right track.

I had an appointment with my GP and told her about the change my hair was experiencing. She looked at me with a smile and said, "Hormones."

What?

"You're going through the change."

Noooo. I'm too young to be going through the change.

"Hormones," she repeated.

She ran through a list of other signs I could be entertaining menopause but I pointed out to her that those symptoms could also be associated with multiple sclerosis. We came to the conclusion that the best thing to do would be to have a blood test done. The test would clearly tell what state my hormones were or weren't in and then we would know for sure whether or not the wavy hair was magic or sputtering hormones. The hormone levels in the blood test were normal. So much for the menopause theory. My hair and I felt vindicated.

My two former bosses included me in the group that was going to Orlando to celebrate the opening of a project they had created there. It was the last project I worked on before I had to leave the development company and I was so flattered and excited to be included in the event. I bought a great sexy sleeveless clinging black crêpe formal with a slit up the side of the leg and a plunging scoop at the back modified by fine black net. It was fabulous.

The hotel we stayed in was very spacious, too spacious for me to get around without a struggle so we rented a wheelchair. We were there for a week. During the day the rest of the group took in the sights around Orlando while I parked myself by the pool and waited for their return. When they got back we went out for dinner. The night of the project opening was warm. There were two orchestras, one at either end of the project site and all of the stores and restaurants in the entertainment center were open for guests to wander through. There was a wonderful spread of food, and tuxedos and sequins were everywhere. I got in and out of my wheelchair as my legs allowed and by the time we got back to the hotel bar to wind up the evening, I was walking just fine.

Sitting at a table talking with friends, one of the men suddenly asked, "Cath, have you been to the bathroom lately?" I was taken aback by the question. He pointed at my hair and said, "You gotta check that out."

So I went to the ladies room and as soon as I caught sight of myself in the humongous wall mirror, I saw Bozo the Clown in a sexy sleeveless clinging black crêpe formal with a slit up the side of the leg. The only time I had seen my hair look like that was once after a bad perm. The climate in Edmonton is dry at an altitude of approximately 2000 feet above sea level. Orlando is humid at sea level. The women in our party who had straight hair spent hours trying to get their flat lifeless hair to respond to any kind of lift in the humid air. My newly wavy hair sprang into tight curls in the sparkling Orlando night.

When I got back to Edmonton I tried various hairdressers to see if I could find one who knew how to handle wavy hair. It wasn't easy and I had a couple of disasters but eventually the person I found worked in a salon directly across the street from where I lived. She was terrific. The shorter we cut it the wavier my hair got. I went out for dinner one night with my friends from the Red Cross and I was sitting in the front seat of the car. One of the ladies sitting in the back seat who was looking at the back of my head said, "What did you do to your hair? Wait. Don't tell me. You washed your hair in the kitchen sink, scrunched it with your hands when it was drying and that's all you did."

"Yup."

"I hate you."

It's good to have friends.

My wavy hair might very well have been the by-product of hormones starting to do the peri-menopause thing and if this was menopause I looked good. I hadn't expected that. I chose to look at my wonderful wavy hair as God's consolation prize. I couldn't dance anymore but I looked good. He had clobbered me with MS, added a generous helping of losses, fear and frustration and He was pretty clear what I thought about it all. I made sure of that. So maybe after all my ranting and cursing He decided to throw me a bone. He knew how hard showering was for me. He saw how pathetic I was trying to handle a blow dryer and a brush at the same time so He decided to give me a break. Maybe He figured – all right, her dance card won't be full but that doesn't mean she can't look pretty sitting on the sidelines, especially if she has colorful streamers in her spokes.

My wavy hair was great. I would never have thought about asking God for something like that. I would never have thought about asking for MS either. I preferred to look at the wavy hair as a sign that all of my efforts and the work I was doing with Dan and Kevin meant I was making progress, incremental though it might be. God couldn't be such a mean piece of work if He could also hand out wavy hair.

God and I weren't exactly on the same page at that point but I have to say I was thinking about Him differently. One of my mother's favourite sayings is 'God is good'. Looking at my wavy hair I thought it could be that our senses of humor were different but if He was willing to give me wavy hair then maybe there were a couple of other things we could work on together, like walking.

Segment 4 – Every Person

Every person,

all the events of your life

are there because you have

drawn them there.

What you choose

to do with them is

up to you.

Richard Bach
Illusions

Mr. Irving

When Dan and Kevin talked about concepts they were introducing to me, intellectually I had no problem following their train of thought. We had terrific conversations. It could take quite a while, however, for those concepts to move beyond intellect to registering with me on an emotional level. Months could go by and then one day I would go into their office excited and joyful that something we had been discussing had finally "hit my bones." With great enthusiasm I would then proceed to explain it all to them. On more than one occasion Dan looked at me and said "What the hell did you think we were talking about?" "I know," I would answer. "But I just got it. It hit my bones this morning while I was brushing my teeth."

After this happened a few times I realized I had a history of learning like this. I could grasp ideas quite easily on an intellectual basis but if I really wanted to understand, truly get hold of an idea, figure out where it started from and how it got to the place where I saw it, it took some time to "hit my bones."

When I was in grade nine, I had a two hour math class every day with Mr. Irving. The first hour of the class he would teach.

The second hour of the class he would tutor us individually as we requested his help or we could do our homework assignments.

My nemesis in grade nine math was the Pythagorean Theorem. That's algebra. Pythagoras was an ancient Greek and centuries later he was making my life miserable. I just didn't understand how he got to that formula for triangles. I could've just memorized the formula and blundered ahead but I really wanted to know how he got there so I could apply it properly to other problems. So every day when Mr. Irving said we could work on whatever math problems or homework we had, I flipped open my math book to the well-worn crease at the beginning of the chapter on good old Pythagoras and tried to understand what his theorem was all about.

Months went by and the struggle continued. I was one of those students who sailed through English, composition (they don't teach that anymore), and other related language arts subjects but math and science were a struggle. I wasn't stupid. I just didn't think that way.

One day when Mr. Irving had given us the signal that we could work on our own math assignments, he looked at me and said, "What are you going to work on, Cathy?" He had a cheeky little know-it-all grin on his face. I flipped open the math book and it landed automatically at the well-creased start of the chapter on the Pythagorean Theorem. I looked down at the page and a moment later made a noise.

Oh.

I heard Mr. Irving say, "Come here." When I looked up, I saw him sitting at his desk holding out a long piece of white chalk to me.

I got up from my desk carefully and walked to the front of the room deliberately. I didn't want to make any sudden moves that would dislodge the fragile ideas being entertained gingerly in my brain. I took the chalk from his hand, went to the blackboard and started to write. When I was done I had filled the entire blackboard at the front of the classroom with the Pythagorean Theorem including triangle drawings.

I stared at the blackboard. I don't think I had taken a breath since I left my desk. The classroom was quiet. Everybody knew I had a mental block where Pythagoras was concerned and here I had just written out his entire theorem from stem to stern on the blackboard for everyone to see. I didn't have to do that. All we needed to know was the last equation based on a triangle and I could have memorized that easily enough but I needed to know how the whole theorem worked.

The next thing I heard was Mr. Irving saying I could go. I had done enough for that day. I went to my desk, picked up my books and left the classroom. I didn't know where to go so I went to the big, empty cafeteria and just sat there by myself. I sat there until the bell rang and I could go to my next class.

A month later, my family moved from Montréal to Calgary. My father had accepted a transfer from the company he worked for to start a branch office in the West. A couple of months after that, we heard the shocking news that Mr. Irving had died in a canoeing accident with another teacher, the teacher my sister had the year before and liked very much. It took awhile for their bodies to turn up but eventually they were recovered from the St. Lawrence River. I guess Mr. Irving and his buddy had had enough for this round.

For years I thought how sad it was that Mr. Irving had spent almost an entire school year just waiting for one student to understand one math equation and then he died. Surely, I could have made his life easier if I had understood that theorem right at the beginning of the school year and we could have moved on from there to other math problems. Instead he got stuck with me and then it was over.

Later on, I began to think that if I had to learn that particular piece of math, he was probably the best teacher to provide me with the time, patience and space I needed. I probably couldn't have done what I did on the blackboard that day with any other teacher. It took him. That's why he was there that year and that's why I was in his classroom. Perhaps my understanding that theorem and being able to write it out on the blackboard from beginning to end was exactly the validation he needed that he was a good teacher. Perhaps I was just exactly the right student for him at that time in his life.

I was very grateful that he had so patiently waited for me to understand it finally. He was a good guy and a good teacher. I guess he knows that teaching me that piece of math was one of the accomplishments of his life and my learning it from him was one of mine. All these years later here I am writing about it and remembering him. And there I was years later in Dan and Kevin's office, finally "getting" an idea after months of their patient repetition. Different lessons, same learning process, new understandings.

A Rider's View

My former boss's wife called me one day and asked if I'd ever thought about riding a horse. *I have multiple sclerosis, for God's sake. I can't take a single unaided step without falling down. Ride a horse? Yeah, right.*

She explained that two of her sisters volunteered at a thing called Little Bits. It was a therapeutic riding program down at the Whitemud Equine Centre. I'd never heard of it and I didn't know such a thing existed in Edmonton. She said there was a class of ladies with MS who rode there. Would I be interested in watching them sometime? Sure I said, why not.

So on a cold, clear November morning we went to the Equine Centre to watch the MS ladies ride. They were very impressive, trotting and turning on the instructor's command. While the class was going on I was introduced to the woman who ran the program and a number of the volunteers who were working that day. When the MS ladies were finished their class, I was introduced to them and we had a chance to talk about their experiences with Little Bits.

The enthusiasm, positive energy and good natured, pure fun was evident in everyone's attitude – from the riders who had various physical and developmental disabilities to the volunteers and family members watching the classes. I decided that day to sign up for the next session in the spring. In April, when I began riding with my own class, I saw that my first impression of Little Bits was real.

As the weather warmed up we moved our classes from inside the arena to the trails along the river. Wonder of wonders, I was back in the river valley. Before my diagnosis I hiked and rode my bike on those trails but hadn't been on them since. I missed them. Now on a beautiful, spring evening I was back in the river valley again. I heard birds singing, hooves clopping on the hard earth, and the laughter and wisecracking remarks of riders, volunteers and instructors as we moved between the trees beside the wonderful North Saskatchewan River. My heart was breathing.

I knew thoroughbreds raced in the Kentucky Derby, Clydesdales pulled the Budweiser wagon, Big Ben leapt over tall jumps and Roy Rogers rode a Palomino named Trigger. I didn't realize until I started riding at Little Bits just how different one horse was from the other in terms of personality. At Little Bits, the horses were older so they were gentler to ride. Pete was a dapple Grey who fell asleep if you stopped for longer than ten seconds during a class. Pax was a Palomino and everyone's favourite. They tried to retire him from the classes when he reached a certain age but he stopped eating. So they saddled him up for class once a day and his appetite and health improved immediately. I got to ride Pax once. He was all business. He had an arch in his neck and he marched with his shoulders bunched up taking one military step after the other. I can't say he was a comfortable ride because when he moved I could feel every bone in that old horse's body. Pax passed away at thirty-six years old. When Tuffy turned forty he made the evening news. Tuffy and I weren't a great partnership. I don't know why in particular except we just didn't seem to be on the same page.

And then they gave me Ribbon to ride. Ribbon was part Arabian. I don't know exactly how old she was but in that elderly group of horses, she was probably among the younger ones. The first night I had her we were getting lessons in how to steer. I was told by one of the volunteers to really pull hard on the rein if I wanted to go right or left and especially if I was going to give Ribbon the signal to back up – pull back hard on the reins until she started to walk in reverse. Every time I pulled hard on the reins, Ribbon retaliated by suddenly tossing her head and wrenching my arms out of their sockets.

When I got back to class the next week and they told me I would be riding Ribbon again, I was not thrilled. When I tried to steer and pull hard on her rein she did the same thing – she suddenly tossed her head so my offending arm got yanked hard straight from the shoulder. I decided to heck with that. I was just going to let her do whatever it was she wanted to do. And then I don't know what I did or how it happened but for some reason I drew the right rein gently up her neck from her shoulder and she instantly turned left. I was stunned. With the left rein I gently drew it up her neck from her shoulder and she immediately turned right. When we were given the command to back up, I held one rein in each hand evenly and gave a tug. She started walking backwards. I thought this is what it must be like to drive a Porsche or other high performance vehicle, so finely tuned you hardly have to touch the controls before it's doing what you just thought about. After I understood that about her, Ribbon and I got on just fine.

She hated being in the middle or at the end of a line of horses. She would start walking a little faster than the rest of the group who were obediently staying in line. Once she had passed them all and was the lead horse she could set her own pace and she was a happy camper. When we went up a hill she traversed the grade zigzagging from one side of the path to the other instead of walking straight up. I let the reins go slack and let her do her thing until we got to the top of the hill. When I wanted to go a little faster all I had to do was sit forward a bit and click my tongue. When I wanted to slow down, I sat back and said whoa.

There was a horse named Buck she didn't like at all. If we got within fifteen or twenty feet of him, Ribbon's ears would go flat to her head. When she did that I would talk nicely to her and ever so carefully steer her away from where he was.

At the end of class we gave our horses carrots to thank them for the ride they had given us. The first time I gave carrots to Ribbon, my mother brought them over to us in a bag. Anytime after that when Ribbon saw my mother sitting in the arena she would turn her head to stare at her as we were walking by as if to say "Did you bring them?" I was the one who fed Ribbon the carrots but she knew where the carrots came from – they came from that lady over there with the bag in her hand.

I became anxious about my car driving skills so I signed up for a class on how to drive using hand controls. I figured I would get my car fitted with hand controls and that way I wouldn't have to worry about how dependable my legs were when switching my feet on the foot pedals. I could keep my car and my independence.

The driving lessons were a disaster because I couldn't get it into my head how those hand controls worked. They were the exact opposite to riding a horse. If I wanted to go faster on Ribbon, I leaned forward. In a car with hand controls, if I wanted to increase my speed I pulled *back* on the lever beside the steering wheel. If I wanted Ribbon to stop, I pulled back on the reins. In a car with hand controls, if I wanted to stop I pushed the lever *forward*. In a car with hand controls, push forward meant stop. Pull back meant go. I kept trying to drive that car with hand controls as if it was a horse, which meant I was doing everything completely opposite to how hand controls are set up. It's a wonder I didn't plow the driving instructor and I into a pole.

So it came down to a choice: I could ride a horse, which made total sense to me, or drive a car with hand controls, which made none. I guess I could've gotten used to hand controls but I decided to park my car in the condo's heated underground garage. After a year I was ready to let it go and sold it to a friend. That made sense.

Dan and Kevin encouraged me with the riding and the benefits of working with a horse. One of the things I remember Dan telling me was that when I was riding, my spine met the horse's spine which in turn distributed my energy down each of the horse's four legs which in turn grounded me to the earth through the horse's hooves. That would give me an incredibly stable base for emulating walking, forward movement. As the horse walked my hips shifted side to side as they would if I was walking myself. That was a great image to keep in my mind when I was riding – my spine met Ribbon's spine, which distributed my energy down her four strong legs and I was grounded. I was safe.

Over time, as my symptoms became more evident, I had to re-arrange and re-learn how to do pretty much every activity or chore I did. With Little Bits, I discovered that riding a horse was a brand new activity I learned to do *after* the MS, not something else I gave up *because* of the MS. By itself that was a tremendous thrill. The bonuses were that riding helped my sense of balance and the muscle strength in my legs and no matter what the disability or why people were there, be they riders, instructors, volunteers or family and friends, there were smiles and accomplishment all around and laughter in those barns. My decision to participate in Little Bits as a rider was supported weekly by the efforts of a large group of people – my parents, friends, and the program volunteers. My parents and I made friends there we looked forward to seeing every week.

I haven't ridden at Little Bits for some time but to this day I am profoundly grateful to the entire Little Bits Therapeutic Riding Association for its commitment to making it possible for me and so many others with disabilities to see the world from the back of a gentle horse on a river valley trail in springtime.

Accountable

I was dusting my bookshelf, making room for the latest hot-off-the press paperbacks I had purchased and admiring my growing collection of New Age philosophy, when two of the books that had been on that shelf for years caught my attention.

I remember the day I was in the mall about to pass a bookstore when I impulsively decided to go in. I needed something. I didn't know what I wanted but I figured I could get it in a book. I was hungry for information, a story I could get lost in, something.

I decided I was going to read every book title in the store until I found it. I started going down the wall that ran the length of the store and I read every title of every book on every shelf I passed from floor to ceiling and back again. When I finished that wall at the back of the store, I turned up the first aisle of bookshelves.

A man who was a bit shorter than I was, stepped in front and blocked my view before I could take a good look at the shelf I faced. He picked a book off the rack and passed it back to me without turning around. "This is what you want," he said. I didn't look at the book. I looked at him. He had brown hair, glasses, a blue sweater over a pale yellow shirt and grey slacks. He was very neat. He didn't look at me and he didn't say anything else. He just held out the paperback for me to take. I took the book from him and a woman at the front of the store called out "Are you done?" "Yes," he said. "I'm coming." And off they went.

I took the man's intrusion as a sign and went to the cashier without doing any more browsing. I put the paperback on the counter without looking at it, and started rummaging through my purse for my wallet. Ringing up the sale, the cashier told me how much my purchase was. She put the book in a bag and handed it to me with the change.

When I got home I sat down on the couch and took the book out of the bag. I looked at the front cover for the first time. It was entitled *Grist for the Mill* by some guy named Ram Dass. *Never heard of him*, I thought to myself. I opened up the book and read the first line – "Welcome to an evening under the breast of the Divine Mother." I shut the book fast, tossed it on the kitchen counter and walked away. "Not ready for that one," I said under my breath.

A couple of days later I picked it up again and got past the first line. When I did, I couldn't put it down. I loved every word. It brimmed with ideas about a belief system that was fascinating. My intellect lapped it up. The short man with the glasses and the blue sweater must have been the answer to my unspoken request to find the right book for me at this time. Maybe he was a messenger. Who knew messengers wore glasses? Ask and it will be handed to you at your local mall. Far out.

Next to *Grist* on my bookshelf was the other old favourite, *Illusions* by Richard Bach. It was given to me by a man I was in love with. He gave it to me because it was a book he had enjoyed and it was subject matter he was interested in. I was tickled that he had given me a gift never mind it was a book whose subject matter meant something to him. This was significant sharing.

The full title of the book was *Illusions – The Adventures of a Reluctant Messiah*. It was a wonderful book filled with wisdom the author wrote for the *Messiah's Handbook* he included in the story. The man I was crazy about wrote an inscription at the front of the book paraphrasing one of the sayings from the *Handbook*. He wrote, "Your only obligation in life is to be true to yourself." It was dated July, 1979. I immediately turned to *Grist for the Mill*. The publication date for the paperback edition I had was June, 1981.

I was diagnosed with MS in 1995.

I flipped through the pages of *Illusions* until I found the full saying in the *Handbook* that the paraphrased inscription had been taken from. And there it was. It read, *"Your only obligation in any lifetime is to be true to yourself. To be true to anyone else or anything else is not only impossible but the mark of a fake messiah."*

Be true to yourself. To thine own self be true. They were well-known phrases that had fluttered past my ears from time to time but now I realized I didn't have a clue how to be true to myself. Where to begin? The logical place to start was to re-read those two wonderful books that had been patiently sitting on my bookshelf for almost twenty years, fifteen plus years before my diagnosis. I was in a different place now, in different circumstances. No doubt I would hear what the books had to say differently than I had on my first read through. They would have a fresh and newly inspired impact on me.

I decided being true to me would be both my purpose and challenge in life. I found it a relief to identify a personal life purpose even though I recognized it wouldn't always be easy for me to do. After all those hours working with Dan and Kevin, I was beginning to get an idea about how much and how often I had given my power away.

Maybe the man who gave me *Illusions* was a messenger, too. Maybe the purpose of the MS was to literally stop me in my tracks. Maybe that's what it took to get my attention.

Stay There

I have a friend who in high school had her own phone in her bedroom. Saturday morning we could call her directly and make plans for the day. On more than one occasion when we arrived at her door to pick her up, we discovered she was either still asleep in bed or had no memory of the phone call. We made it a rule that whichever one of our group called her Saturday morning, would redirect the conversation at some point by asking her, "What's your middle name?" The question was unexpected and would wake her up. There would be a bit of a pause on the phone followed by the sound of a quick intake of breath and then her sluggish voice asking, "Who is this?" That's when we knew she was really awake and we had her attention.

Dan and Kevin had the same kind of prompt that they used on me. Whenever we were talking about something and they could see my mind wandering away, they would say, "Stay there." That would always get my attention and my intelligent response was usually something like, "What?"

Dan described my wandering mind as 'pulling out of myself', getting away from me physically. For whatever reason, if I was uncomfortable with the topic of discussion, I would simply wander off in my mind to something that was more pleasant. When either Dan or Kevin saw that happening they would stop me with "Stay there." That would force me back to the subject at hand and make me focus on what we were talking about. When this first started happening, I was unaware that my mind had wandered off but soon I started to recognize when it was about to drift away. I would close my eyes so I could concentrate better and I would ask them to repeat what they had just said over and over until it stuck. Generally speaking, it would take three repetitions before I could repeat it back to them as a sign that I heard what they said. Whether or not I understood the point they were making was a separate issue.

Doofus Angel

He was in our condo working on the windows in the sunroom. The condominium's window replacement saga was finally coming to an end. Five of the six windows in our unit that had to be re-done were in the sunroom where my computer was set up. I was working from home for the marketing department of an engineering company. Needless to say, my ability to work had been severely compromised during the six weeks of construction chaos. I was working at night when the guys doing the window replacement were out of there. I was working at my computer by the light of one lamp that was still plugged in. I was determined those construction doofuses weren't getting in the way of my earning a living anymore, so the morning the interior window trim was being done, I parked myself at the computer. The doofus doing the trim could work around *me* for a change.

It was the first time this guy had been in the condo. The regular crew had finished installing the new windows and had gone. This guy was working alone on the interior window trim that would finish the job. I guessed he was in his early thirties. He kept his yellow wool toque on over his curly shoulder length hair that looked as though it hadn't been combed for days.

I don't know how it started, but within minutes of the two of us being in the same room, we were talking, and the subject matter was heavy from the get-go. He wasn't raised with any religious background he said, but a few years ago, things happened to a buddy of his and he figured he should check out faith and God and Jesus and see what they were all about. But when you don't have a background in those kinds of things, where do you start? He decided to read the Bible and see what it had to say. He'd been studying it ever since.

He liked to study, learn new things. Did I read the Bible? What did I think of Jesus? Did I pray? What is God's law? When I prayed, what did I pray to? He was reading C.S. Lewis' *Pilgrim's Regress*. Had I read that? Did I know *Pilgrim's Progress*? Albert Einstein is an amazing man. Did I know anything about him? Did I know what the implications of the theory of relativity were? The theory of relativity means we can travel at the speed of light, which means we can time travel. But we can't do that yet. You know why? Because we're not the right kind of human being yet. We have to evolve some more before we can take *that* on.

He was teaching himself Greek. So far all he'd learned was the alphabet and if he had known when he started how hard it was, he'd have had second thoughts about learning that language.

He had another construction related company.

Did I do books? He's looking for someone who could do books.

He usually supervises jobs like this one. If they call him to work on a crew, he knows something on the job has gone wrong.

He had an idea for an Internet company. He's taking a business course.

What did I believe in? Did I have any idea what Jesus meant by 'I Am'? Well, this is what he's figured out – because it says in St. Paul – did I know who St. Paul was?

Saul on the road to Damascus.

Yeah, that's the guy. Well, he said, I think it means –

We talked like that all day long, from 8:30 in the morning to 3 in the afternoon with a half-hour break for lunch. I loved it. Every time I looked at this guy he always had his back to me. I only caught sight of his eyes once. Every time I looked at him I thought – *huh?*

He didn't look at all like what he was. This stuff kept spilling out of his mind. There he was, in our condo, in my "office", no one else around and the topics were flying thick and fast. The topics were ones I was interested in, primarily spiritual in nature. He stopped me up a few times with his questions because it would never have occurred to me to think about them. When I instinctively knew what my answer was, I had never said it out loud before. But I knew it was okay to say such things out loud to this guy. In some instances it was the first time I had ever had to create vocabulary about a feeling. I stopped him in his tracks a few times, too. My mother popped her head into the room a couple of times to mouth to me "Okay?" She knew we were talking, but she couldn't hear what we were saying. We both shut up when she popped in.

I was tired by the time he left. He said he'd be back the next day to finish off the last bit of painting that needed to be done. I figured he wanted to continue the conversation but I didn't know how much strength I'd have left. As it turned out, he didn't come back till 3 p.m. the next day. He was wearing a walkman with the earphones on his head on top of the yellow toque, slightly askew so he could still hear what was being said. I heard the music he was playing. "Natalie Merchant, Wonder, Tigerlilly," I said. "I have that tape." "Yeah, great music," he said. He took the walkman off, flipped the tape to the other side, lined it up and handed it to me with the earphones. "Do you know this group?" He had to get some painter's tape. He'd be right back.

I put the earphones on and heard these gorgeous female vices singing Gregorian chant. I almost fell off the chair. What was this guy doing on a work site replacing windows with music like that? He should have had Pearl Jam flailing his eardrums.

Who is this guy?

When he came back and we were talking about the music, I really looked at him. If he lost the yellow cap and combed his hair, he could be quite attractive.

Later, when I described him to Dan, his response was, "You get the people you need when you need them." I said he didn't look anything like what he was. Dan said, "I could say that about some people I know." I ducked because that shot was meant for me. Kevin said "He probably smokes cigarettes, drinks beer and farts", a reference to John Travolta's character Michael in the movie of the same name. He said, "Did you get his number? Did you give him yours? This could be the guy."

Maybe it's like Dan said, I needed someone like him right now to make me organize my thoughts so I could say out loud what I believe. Maybe it was my time to verbalize. Pulling those concepts out of thin air and turning them into vocabulary was a lot of work. It was also fascinating to hear what was coming out of my mouth speaking to a total stranger. Maybe the fact that he was someone I didn't know made it easier to speak.

I guess I was ready for somebody like him to put me through my paces and the Universe provided. I said thank you to both.

"The Edifice of the Dream"

All those weekly trips to the chiropractic clinic, all the therapy, talk, learning, trying, effort and struggle must have been starting to make sense for me. The most recent topic Dan talked to me about was the box that I was in. I wasn't even aware I was in a box but as Dan talked, supported by the work Kevin was doing, I started to hear what they were saying.

Dan pointed out that the rules I was living by for the most part, came from somewhere else. The ideas I heard that I interpreted as rules for how to live or what was expected from me happened early on and came from parents, school, church and my friends when we compared notes playing on the same swing set. Some of those rules I adopted and held as absolute. I used those rules to build my life and created my box.

I wasn't really aware how much I had boxed myself in with my thinking and my beliefs. Not only wasn't I aware but it hadn't dawned on me either that I didn't even like some of those rules I was holding on to so rigidly. Going a step further, it hadn't crossed my mind that I could change my thinking and subsequently change the rules.

Every time I felt angry, every time I seethed with frustration, every time I told myself that the good things in life weren't meant for me, I reinforced the six sides of that box. I think I knew instinctively that this wasn't a good way to live but I was honestly completely clueless about what to do to change it.

Talking with Dan, I was beginning to get a sense of the boxed-in ideas I was living with and how those impenetrable six sides that made up that box came to be. If I understood that I was trapped inside a box I had created; that the box was built from ideas and beliefs I had heard and taken from other people; that some of those ideas and beliefs were skewed or not the right ones for who I was; if I came to understand that, changed my thinking and escaped the box, where would I be? What would I do? How would I handle it? I pictured myself sitting on top of the box looking around but not knowing what to do next. Escape equaled the unknown and courage wasn't my strong suit. It was safer to stay inside the box even if I didn't like it.

The 'box' discussions were still floating around In my head when I came home from work one afternoon to find my copy of the Fifth Agreement Newsletter in my mailbox. Don Miguel Ruiz, author of *The Four Agreements*, had his own column in the newsletter and I usually read that first. His column that month was entitled *Edifice of the Dream*. In it he wrote—

"When you were a baby, your attention was focused in the movement of your muscles until it became automatic. When you learned to walk your attention was in walking. When you learned to speak your attention was in learning the language until it became automatic. When you observed every concept, every action and reaction of the adults around you, you learned from their reactions, more than from their words. And you learned to be the way they are. You learned to be as important as they were, to gossip the way they did, to make everybody else wrong. You learned and you believed that is what you are."

Who wrote this?

I checked the top of the article. It said Don not Dan. The column continued:

"This is not what you are. But by using your attention you put brick on top of brick until you created the whole structure of your dream. That dream is jail, a little box with the real you inside it, and the dream has total control over you."

Did Dan get this newsletter, too? Did he get it before I did and just repeated the ideas back to me? What else does it say?

"... The human form is not the form of your body. No, it's the form of the edifice of your dream, including your name, your identity, your beliefs, your hopes, the image of perfection that you have, all of the lies that you use to dream the dream of your life because every brick that you have is not true. It's a lie."

Oh wow... I don't believe this...

"...You master jealousy, anger, sadness, and gossiping. You master it because you practice it for so many years and you do it perfectly... We no longer want to be so right and make everybody else wrong. We no longer want to judge ourselves or blame ourselves or be guilty, or to be ashamed of ourselves especially when we have the awareness that it's just a dream and it's not Truth."

Oh wow...

"We rebel and we want to change it but wanting to change it doesn't mean that we can change it."

No. Don't tell me that.

"We have created a structure so rigid and so strong. Every habit, every routine, every agreement that we build, every belief, every concept, is so strong that even if our reason understands that it's not healthy for us to function this way, even if our reason understands that we don't want to be that way anymore, it looks hopeless to try to change it."

I know. That's where I am.

"We have mastered our dream so well that changing it becomes difficult. This is because what we have now makes us feel safe, even if we are not happy."

Yes, oh my God, I know.

I was floored. It was Mr. Irving's class all over again and I just got Pythagoras. I got a glass of water. It was as if Dan and Kevin had done all the heavy lifting getting me to a place where I could pick up this newsletter, read Don Miguel's words and know them in my bones. Not only was this newsletter addressed to me, it was written *for* me.

"The only way to change it..." Don Miguel continued.

Great. This is what I need to know.

"... is to use the same tools that we used to build it in the first place... our attention. Every brick that you remove and unlearn, you recover the power that you used to put that brick in the structure in the first place."

Run that by me again.

"It was true that when you were a child you didn't have the opportunity to choose your beliefs, to choose any of the bricks of the building. But this is no longer true. You have the awareness now and you can learn to use your attention for the second time, and have the opportunity to undo your whole structure, to unlearn the whole program, and to choose what you want to believe and create a totally different structure or no structure at all.

Oh wow...

We call this the dream of the second attention because you use your attention for the second time and totally change everything you believe about yourself and your world. The dream of the second attention is the same dream of our everyday life, but a dream where you control the bricks, not where the bricks control you."

Okay. I get that. I control the bricks.

"... there are no limits... you begin to really live for the first time out of the box...

Okay...

"Your whole dream, your whole life, the whole structure that makes you feel so safe is your own jail and it's not even real...When you are alone, you use your own bricks to judge what you feel and what you think. Then we believe in winners and losers. .."

That's the Inside Me.

"Every time that we judge another we are being hypocrites. When you have awareness and realize that this is just a dream, you can finally see the bricks of your dream...Of course, the process of losing the human form is painful."

Is that why I have MS?

"It's painful only because the bricks of the first attention are made of the emotional pain and emotional poison that we have accumulated... Of course, your dream of the first attention has had great and beautiful moments for sure, but it is not my choice to live there. I choose to dream the dream of... what I call the dream of light because we are light and you can learn to dream the way light dreams."

Light dreams? Far out. I am light and I can learn to dream the way light dreams.

"The challenge is to wake up, choose what to believe and become free of your conditioning. Are you ready for the challenge of your life?"

Well, I guess I must be because I'm reading this newsletter.

Dan and Kevin are singing the same tune. I can change this. Don Miguel said all we had to do was be aware of the bricks, what they are made of and change them.

Great. Change them to what?

And then there's still the question of when I get outside the box. Can I be brave enough to give up a safe place even if I don't like it? Should I know what I want to do before I get out of the box? Should I be making a ten year plan? Where do I want to be in ten years? Where do I want to be in five? I hate ten year plans. I hate goal setting because I don't know what the goals are or what they should be. I've always felt I had to have all the answers instantly. I learned that from my father. He always had the answers. Well, I definitely don't have all the answers right now so if I start to climb out of the box before having all the answers, will that make me an adventurer or an idiot?

"The challenge is to wake up."

Okay. I'm awake but would it be okay if after I get out of the box I just kind of, you know, hung around for a bit, let my wings dry in the sun until I'm ready to, you know, do something. Would that be okay?

And Then There Is Simply a Gift

In November, 1997 I flew home from Orlando where I had spent a week attending the grand opening of the last commercial real estate project I was involved with before I had to stop working full time. The MS had taken its toll and I was too tired and weak to work full-time anymore especially at the pace I had been keeping. I was thrilled when some months after I left the company my former bosses included me in the trip to Orlando to see our largest project to date completed and open for business.

On the trip home to Edmonton I stopped in Minneapolis to change planes. Minneapolis has a big airport so I used one of the terminal carts to move from one gate to the next. At the gate for my connecting flight to Edmonton I transferred to an airport wheelchair, which made it easier for the airline staff to move me from the gate to the plane. I boarded the aircraft along with mothers with small children. I used my cane to hobble down the aisle to my seat in Row 18, seat A by the window. When those of us who needed extra time and assistance were settled, the rest of the passengers were allowed to board.

On the side of the plane where I was sitting each row had two seats. On the other side of the aisle the rows had three seats. From the crowd of people pushing past each other in the narrow aisle, a fellow sat down in the seat beside me. We were going to be sitting beside each other for the next three hours and whether or not we ever said another word to one another, I thought a simple hello was in order. Before I could say anything he stood up again. I watched him take his leather jacket off and stuff it into the overhead bin. I watched him because his looks reminded me of a type of guy I had met before. And then it hit me. I knew exactly who he was.

We met at university. I was 18. He was two years older. We had three rounds in eight years. That's what I called it. He was there, we were together, then he left. He was there, we were together, then he left again. He was there, we were together, and as I recall I was the one who left that third time. I remember getting out of his car and saying "Call me in three years." I slammed the car door shut and walked away. I cried and cried and cried. Why couldn't we make this work?

Towards the end of round three we were at his company's Christmas party and I met his co-workers for the first time. They had no idea we had the lengthy history that we did and they welcomed me with open arms like I was his new girlfriend. We were having a great time. I remember being in the kitchen talking to some people and looking out towards the living room where he was standing. He was in great spirits and laughing. We were happy, having fun, being the best we could be.

It's not enough.

That's what went across my mind as I watched him. What a shocking thought. We were having a wonderful time, it was Christmas, we loved each other and yet in that moment I knew it wasn't enough. I always thought if you loved somebody enough your relationship could handle anything. But standing there in that cheerful fun crowd anticipating Christmas holidays, I realized for all the history we had and all we had been through with each other, the love that we felt wasn't enough. It wasn't enough to succeed. It wasn't enough for a happy ending or the beginning of a long life together. I loved him. I had loved him for so long. There he was in the living room laughing and about as attractive as I had ever seen him and all the love I felt wasn't enough. The relationship didn't end that night but it wasn't too long afterwards that it did. Now twenty years later, there he was folding his leather jacket, stuffing it into the overhead bin on this Northwest Airlines plane headed for Edmonton, headed home, and he was sitting beside me.

You know those car chases in Los Angeles you see on TV being followed from helicopters? Police cars pursue the suspect driving like a maniac down a freeway dodging slower moving vehicles until – *bam*. It smashes into some poor car dawdling through an intersection. No matter how many times I see that piece of film I'm always startled when the two vehicles collide. I looked at the man standing in the aisle innocently folding his jacket and reaching for the overhead bin, not for a second being aware that a past-life-collision was about to happen. He was about to get broadsided and he didn't know it. I knew it was going to happen, I just didn't know the exact moment when he would know it. I knew and that knowledge came with a wonderful empowering feeling. That must be how God feels sometimes looking at us.

He sat down beside me and I looked at him with a big grin on my face. I couldn't help it. He glanced at me, nodded and looked away. I kept staring and grinning. He glanced at me again, nodded and started to go through the seat pocket in front of him looking for something to read. I kept staring and grinning. I was determined not to say anything until I saw the light of recognition cross his eyes. When he looked at me the third time his face said "Lady, what is your problem?" I just stared and grinned. And then I saw it, the light of recognition.

Bam.

I saw his eyesight clear. He turned his head slightly and said "Cassie?" I said 'hi' and we both burst out laughing. When we regained our composure he said "So, what have you been doing for the last twenty years?"

We didn't reminisce. We got caught up on where our lives were now. We filled three hours talking without going backwards or running out of things to say. At one point I excused myself to go to the washroom. On the way back to my seat I stopped by a coworker who had also attended the project opening in Orlando. I said to her, "See that man I'm sitting beside?" She said yes and then I said, "I could have married him twenty years ago" and continued walking back to my seat. It was important to me that someone witnessed this astounding event happening in Row 18, seats A and B.

As the plane descended into Edmonton, he said two things that I didn't realize until he said them that I needed to hear. The first thing he said was that he had thought about me from time to time over the years and wondered how I was doing. I had thought the same thing about him, too, but I always figured that for him I was out of sight and out of mind. It turns out I wasn't. I was surprised and pleased to hear that every now and then we both wondered how the other was doing.

The second thing he said was in relation to the MS. He said I had a good attitude about it and he added "but then you always did have a good attitude." That was news to me coming from him. I remember him calling me 'childish' on more than one occasion so to hear he thought I had a good attitude was remarkable personal validation.

Isn't the Universe breathtaking? Twenty years after the fact it gives me an airplane ticket for Row 18 Seat A by the window and it gives him a ticket for Row 18 Seat B on the aisle. I came from Orlando to connect with that plane. He travelled from somewhere else he'd been on business. The Universe put us at 33,000 feet for three hours. We could have ignored each other but we didn't. Once upon a time we loved each other.

We got caught up on who we were now, dickered for the lousy little lunch they served us, and we laughed. I came away from that flight feeling gratitude and forgiveness. I forgave him and I forgave me. When I got off the plane, I felt an overwhelming sense of peace the likes of which I had never felt before nor have I felt since.

I must be on track.

Be well, old friend, wherever you are.

Segment 5 – Go Deeper

When one thinks -

"Now I have touched the bottom of the sea,

now I can go no deeper,"

one goes deeper.

Katherine Mansfield

The Red Pill or the Blue Pill

Kevin started the session by holding out his closed hands to me asking if I wanted to take the red pill – he opened one hand – or the blue one – he opened the other hand. When he opened his hands, they were empty.

"What?"

"Do you want to take the red pill or the blue one?" He did the same closed, open movements with his hands.

"I have no idea what you're talking about."

"Have you seen The Matrix?"

"No."

"Why not?"

"Because it's just a lot of shooting guns."

"Who said that?"

"Nobody. It's the TV ads."

"You gotta see it."

The movie left the theatres and after more prodding from Kevin, I went to Blockbuster and rented it.

When the movie got to the scene where Morpheus offers Neo his choice of taking a red pill or a blue one, I understood what it was Kevin wanted to know. Morpheus explained to Neo that if he chose the blue pill he would wake up the next day with no memory of having met Morpheus and life would go back to what it was, the man known as John Anderson (Neo) working for the agents in a mundane office job. If Neo chose to take the red pill it would be his trip down the rabbit hole to a life he couldn't begin to imagine.

The answer to Kevin's question was I would take the red pill. I figured I had already taken it. I took it the day I drove out of the good doctor's parking lot and never went back. The basement chiropractic clinic was probably the rabbit hole. When I drove out of that parking lot I took the red pill, went down the rabbit hole and found Dan and Kevin, not exactly mainstream. The next appointment I had with Kevin, I went into his office and said, "The red pill." He grinned. I haven't looked at a box of Smarties the same way since.

Emotional Coward

A first cousin of my father's came out west with his family for a holiday one summer. For some reason his wife asked my mother about me while I was standing right there. My mother delivered the most shocking description of me I had ever heard. My mother said I was a good person but "not very honest." I didn't ask her what she meant by that nor did I react in any way. I was so shocked by the description that I just stood there dumbfounded. I thought she was completely out to lunch and thoroughly resented her remark but the description stuck with me for years.

It wasn't until I started doing the work to find out what had got me in this multiple sclerosis pickle that I remembered her remark. When I thought about it in terms of my medical predicament, I realized she was right. I wasn't very honest. I was honest about things like filing my income tax or doing my job but I was not honest about my feelings with others or more importantly, with myself. In fact, I realized there were two me's. There was what I thought of as the *inside me* and there was an *outside me*.

The outside me was the person I presented for the world to see. The outside me was the mask. The inside me gave new meaning to low self-esteem. I wallowed in it. I was scared to death that one day I would be exposed for the miserable excuse of a person I believed I was. I was so not-good-enough it was breathtaking. This discrepancy between what I saw as the outside me and what I knew was the inside me meant that I was always in survival mode, just barely getting by. When I felt safe in a situation or safe with the people I was with it wasn't as bad. But I always felt the fear and trying to hold off the threat of exposure kept my brains occupied every minute of every day.

It takes a humongous amount of effort and energy to hold the world at bay.

Fear of Being Vulnerable

I have a paralyzing Fear of being vulnerable.

I avoid being vulnerable by not expressing who I am.

When I don't express who I am, I empower my Fear.

When I give my power away to my Fear,

My life becomes an expression of that Fear.

Reflections on the Negative Stew

Did the inside-me and the outside-me line up? Were they in sync? Did they reflect each other or were they opposites? If they were opposed to each other, would they eventually line up? What was the inside-me filled with? It was filled with anger, self-pity and hurt. Were they real or imagined? Did it matter? Did I nurse the negativity allowing it to fester? Was the persona that I presented to the world, the outside-me, as capable, efficient and managing life as well as I thought I was? Was the inside-me the negative stew that fuelled the MS? Was the negative stew reflected in the outside-me? What fuelled the negative stew? What gave the negative stew the energy it needed to reflect itself as disease in the outside-me?

What did I know? I knew about the negativity. What could I do about that? I could stop it. How? Just stop it. When I hear myself having those negative conversations with myself over and over and over again, just stop it. Think about something else. Do something. Every time my thoughts drift back into their old miserable habits, stop and change direction. Will it change the fact that I have MS? No. But could it make it better? Yes. I believe that.

I had to start some where. Like the *Messiah's Handbook* said, to mine own self be true. That was my job. That's what I had to do. That's what I had to figure out. That's why I'm here.

This is no longer a choice.

Addicted to Feeling Bad

I was so angry. I don't know when the anger started or how long it had been going on. It just seemed that was the way things were in my emotional world: angry. I focused my anger on work because that was the biggest part of my life and I played out the angry work-related scenarios in my mind constantly. I wasn't married. I hadn't even had a boyfriend in ages. I didn't belong to any wonderfully interesting organizations or volunteered regularly for any civic events or charities. Work was my life; that and spending time with friends.

So I replayed the office injustices in my head over and over and over. The angry office playlists could be based on something somebody said that day or a task I didn't particularly like doing or maybe having to deal with someone I didn't get along with. It would be something of that nature. I starred in my mind-movie as the righteous martyr victim and "they" were the evil, mean, protagonists bent on making my life hell. The cast of characters for who "they" were changed a little bit in terms of who was the lead character in the anger scenario at the moment. Every time I played the situation over in my head, I adjusted the dialogue a little bit here, a little bit there to benefit my role as righteous martyr heroine. I always got the best lines, the fabulous putdowns, the stunning self-righteous declarations that would stun and mesmerize my opponents. My power remarks were second to none. I couldn't stop hitting the repeat button so the nasty movie just kept playing over and over and over. The reruns didn't stop and the truth is there was a large part of me that didn't want to stop them.

I would have been lost if I didn't feel bad every day. I craved the negative emotional hit my brain gave me. I was like a junkie getting my dose of angry-martyr-victim in the safety and solitude of my own mind. I didn't see it that way at the time. In fact, I didn't see it at all.

The MS diagnosis could have brought an entirely new facet to my victim mind-movie but it didn't. Instead of incorporating the diagnosis into my existing martyr playback and coming up with something incredibly miserable, I thought of the play going on in my mind and the diagnosis as separate things. I could have been profoundly content to wallow in my miserable seething martyrdom and add all the implications of that shocking diagnosis to my victim repertoire but for some reason I didn't.

The doctors didn't know where MS came from, how it started, how to prevent it, how to treat it, and improving the condition was a very iffy proposition left only to the imaginings of alternative medicine practitioners. I was trapped in an unknown disease whose prognosis was the definition of bleak. My future was spiraling downwards at what was predicted to be a pretty fast clip. And yet I didn't include MS in my anger. I was angry at the helpless doctors and I was angry at my body for its deliberate yet bewildering betrayal.

In my sessions with Dan and Kevin it came out that I was addicted to feeling bad. Running angry scenarios over and over in my mind wasn't just a bad habit. I was addicted to it. I was addicted to running the scenarios because I was addicted to feeling the anguish of the martyr victim. I enjoyed it. I created it. What a concept. I was so used to running the anger scenes and dialogue repeatedly in my head that I didn't see them or hear them. It was so much a part of me, feeling angry at the world and bad about myself, that it was my state of normal.

Dan and Kevin identifying this need for twisted thinking as an addiction so I could give myself an emotional high, gave me the opportunity to observe myself doing it. It was a tremendous break-through for me.

I looked up Louise Hay to see what she had to say about addic-tions. She said the probable cause for addictions is running from the self. Fear. Not knowing how to love the self. Well, that was certainly true for me.

The next question I asked myself was how do I get rid of this addiction? After I thought about it, I realized I had not only experi-enced addiction before, I had successfully conquered it. I had quit smoking. I smoked cigarettes for sixteen years. Not a small accom-plishment. I had beaten the addiction ten years earlier. If I had overcome that addiction then I knew I could overcome the addiction to feeling bad. I just needed to remember how I had quit smoking and figure out how to apply that successful strategy to healing an emotional appetite for negative stew.

How I Quit Smoking

I quit smoking on my thirty-fifth birthday. I didn't plan it that way. No, wait a minute. That's not exactly correct. I had been trying to quit for about a year. The cost of a package of cigarettes had gone up to $2.25. (Does anyone remember that far back?) I thought that was an outrageous price and I wasn't going to pay it. So that was my incentive to quit.

A friend purchased a little book about how to quit smoking. It was helpful but we got the how-to-quit package from the Canadian Lung Association and that was better. They had all kinds of suggestions for how to go about monitoring when, how many and why we smoked. It took the better part of a year but by using their method I cut back from a pack to five cigarettes a day. That was great but I couldn't seem to get below five. I had it in my mind that when I cut back consistently to two or three cigarettes a day then I would be able to flat out quit. But I got to five cigarettes a day and plateaued there.

I woke up on my thirty-fifth birthday feeling like I might be coming down with a cold. At work, people wished me happy birthday and asked if I would be going out that night to celebrate. I said no, I felt like I was getting a cold, and I wanted to beat it before it got ahead of me. The party was going to be in Jasper on Saturday and I didn't want to miss it. I had a friend there who shared the same birth date, although different years. We had been celebrating our birthdays together since we met at university. The party was sometimes where I lived and sometimes where he lived. This year it was going to be at his place in Jasper.

After dinner, I curled up on the couch under a blanket with my cigarettes on the end table beside me. I spent the evening answering phone calls from family and friends wishing me happy birthday. It was fun and I was glad I was home.

When I woke up the next morning I knew immediately I was in trouble. My chest felt heavy and bruised and when I went to make a sound it was like a seal with the croup. I phoned my doctor's office and left a message on their answering machine that I needed to see the doctor if she had some time that day. I have no idea how I got that message out or what it must have sounded like on the other end. When I phoned my company office to let them know I wouldn't be in, it took three tries before the receptionist stopped hanging up on me and realized who was calling.

The doctor's office phoned back and said they had time to see me that morning. I called a cab because I knew I couldn't drive. I felt so lousy. When I got to the doctor's office she asked me how I was and I made that seal-with-the-croup noise. She asked me what hurt and with my hand I indicated from my chin to my belly button. After her exam, she declared that I had a respiratory tract infection and my temperature was 102°. No wonder I didn't want to drive. I was practically delirious. She prescribed medication and told me I should also buy a cold water humidifier to help with my breathing.

The pharmacist was a young Chinese man who rushed around and got everything I needed including an extra box of Kleenex. I must have looked bad. Using a combination of hand signals and my croupy seal voice, he called a cab for me and helped me out with my purchases.

Back home I fell into a deep sleep on the couch bundled under my favourite blanket. Each time I woke up I took my temperature and each time it had risen by another hash mark on the thermometer. My mother called in the afternoon. She had phoned the office and found out I was sick and hadn't come to work that day. She came over a little later and I gave her some money to buy me soup. In between her coming and going I fell asleep. Each time I woke up I took my temperature again. When it got to one hash mark under 103°, I thought the next time I wake up, if my temperature is right on 103°, I'm going to emergency. But it didn't move up to 103°. It was still sitting at that hash mark when I crawled off to bed for the night.

The next morning I woke up when my mother walked into the bedroom. My parents had the spare key to my apartment and she wanted to know how I was doing. All I could tell her was how sore I felt from head to toe. Every part of me ached. The fever had broken overnight, which was good, but I didn't feel like I had any strength at all. I spent most of that day in bed sleeping and any time I did get up to go to the bathroom or make myself something to eat, my temperature immediately shot back up to 101°. Needless to say, I didn't get to Jasper.

The third day I felt well enough to sit on the couch again. When I walked into the living room I saw my package of cigarettes lying on the end table where I'd left them two nights earlier. I realized I hadn't had a cigarette in that time and I sure hadn't missed them. So I picked up the package, walked into the kitchen and threw it in the garbage pail under the sink. And that was that.

When I got back to the office on Monday, I told people I hadn't had a cigarette now for five days and I didn't feel like having one at all. One of the older ladies, who was an avid proponent of smoking, insisted that I have one of her cigarettes. She wouldn't take no for an answer and I was curious about how it would feel to have a cigarette again after five days without one. I took her cigarette and lit it. I haven't tasted anything quite that awful since. It was probably the medication I was taking that altered my taste buds but I didn't try smoking a cigarette again for a while. I'm not sure how long after that awful tasting experience, I did go out and buy a package of cigarettes for some reason. I had smoked about half of it when I realized what I was doing. *Stupid.*

I threw the rest of the package away and never smoked again.

Sixteen years I smoked. For the better part of one year I actively worked at quitting my addiction and cut back from one pack to five single cigarettes a day. In the end, it was a respiratory tract infection and a 103° temperature that did the job. Now I could have a coffee, talk on the phone, drive my car, have a heart-to-heart discussion with a friend, and I never missed having a cigarette in my hand. I didn't crave the nicotine. I chalked that up to the fact that I had had such a high fever. I figured it had burned out every last bit of nicotine that had been hiding in my body including that obscure cell waiting for just the right moment to pounce on my central nervous system and reactivate the craving. Thank God for 103° temperatures.

Now I had to figure out how to stop being addicted to feeling bad. I could use the example that the Canadian Lung Association outlined in its material -- become aware of when, how many, and why I reached for a cigarette. I would have to become aware of when, how often and why I ran those angry movies in my mind where I was the victimized heroine. I could use those how to quit smoking techniques to learn how to stop running those angry movies in my mind. See, I was thinking if the 103° fever burned the nicotine out of every cell in my body so I could quit smoking, then maybe if I figured out how to clear every cell of the need to feel bad then that could clear every cell of the MS. It was a way to start.

One Opportunity at a Time

When I hear a song I like and I don't hum along,

I suppress my joy.

When I write with hesitation, I suppress my gift.

When I don't express my love

either in word or deed,

I deaden my heart and disappoint my spirit

one opportunity at a time.

Expectations

What Mothers Do

Mothers feed you when you're hungry. They pick you up and dust you off when you trip. They listen to your stories and laugh at your silly jokes. They find answers for your questions and suggest solutions for your problems. They fix things. They are there and they are always pitching even if you don't like the ball they're throwing. They are your best audience. They are your best critics. They are on your side.

I know there are people out there whose mothers weren't what they hoped they would be but that wasn't my experience, thank goodness. On more than one occasion I fell walking from the bathroom to the bedroom on my way to bed. My mother would size up the situation and figure out a way to get me back up and on my bed. She came up with an ingenious plan where she took the cushions from the living room couch and one at a time got them underneath me. Each time I was raised a little bit higher. I got from the floor to my knees and my feet and onto the bed with one last lift effort from her.

The exacerbation I had that landed me in a wheelchair happened just as suddenly as the exacerbation that put me on a cane. It was a matter of a couple of days from when I first felt something wasn't right until I had to use equipment. My father rented the wheelchair and I needed it. There was no way around the fact that I couldn't walk.

I was devastated.

I have cried that hard twice in my life and that was the second time. I got into bed and I couldn't stop myself. When a day had taken its toll, I tried to do my crying between midnight and 6 a.m. I hoped my parents wouldn't hear me and I could get the disappointment out of my system before I had to face another day and pretend that I was fine. Maybe I was the only one who was trying to fool me but that night the tears flowed.

I didn't try to whimper or keep it to myself. I sobbed. How could this be happening to me? Why did I have this horrible, miserable, disease? I had found two of the best people I've ever met who worked with me whenever I called, whenever I showed up. Thanks to their patience I was learning things, I understood things about myself for the first time; so how could this be happening? How could I be getting worse? When would it stop? Would it only stop like the medical establishment said, when I was virtually a vegetable in a bed in a long-term care facility waiting for the end? Was that all I had dreamed for myself, hoped for myself in this lifetime?

Come on, God. Make it stop.

When I couldn't think anymore, when breathing was just a series of sobs I couldn't control, that's when my mother laid down on the bed beside me. She didn't try to hug me or hold my hand. She didn't try to talk to me. She couldn't kiss it and make it better. She couldn't make it go away but she could be there. She could be my company, my companion in sorrow. She lay on the bed beside me so I wasn't alone. I don't remember when I finally fell asleep. I don't remember when she went to her own room. I do know she got less sleep than I did that night. That's what a mother does. That's what my mother did.

Segment 6 – God Builds Its Temple

God builds its temple

in the heart

on the ruins of churches and religions.

Ralph Waldo Emerson

In Order to Be Whole
and Complete

Dan figured it out. He said, "You suffer in order to be whole and complete."

"What was that?"

"In order for you to be whole and complete, you believe you have to suffer."

"Run that one by me again."

"When you're suffering, that's when you believe you're whole and complete."

"As long as I'm suffering, I think I'm whole and complete?'

"Right."

"I have MS so that means I'm suffering?"

"Right."

"So, as long as I have MS I think I'm whole and complete?"

"Right."

"If I didn't have MS, if I was healthy, I wouldn't be whole and complete?"

"You believe you have to suffer first."

"So I am a whole and complete person as long as I have MS?"

"Right."

"That doesn't make any sense. Why would I do that to myself?"

"It doesn't matter. That's what you believe."

"Wow..."

In discussions with Dan about the nature of my MS, he surmised that in order for me to be a whole and complete person I believed I had to suffer.

The first thing I thought of was being Catholic. His description of me as a personality fit with what he said. I always understood that in order to be a good Catholic meant there was a fundamental need to suffer. I was taught that we are imperfect human beings. We commit sins. Not only do we commit sins, we come into this life with our souls already spoiled with sin. We are born with Original Sin.

If we die while our souls are stained with sins, we go to Purgatory or we go to hell depending on the severity of our sins. We redeem ourselves by going to confession where we wipe the slate clean, so to speak, until we commit our next sins and so repeat the cycle.

The most readily available suffering a Catholic can do is to sacrifice. When I was a kid and Lent came around, making a sacrifice meant maybe I gave up eating candy or watching my favourite TV show until Lent was over. One of my father's favourite expressions when he was doing without something was "I'm offering it up." It was said as a joke, not piously.

The ultimate sacrifice is martyrdom. Suffering, sacrifice and martyrdom are applauded and encouraged by the church that's trying to save my wretched soul. For those things, I was taught, I would be rewarded. If I didn't suffer, my eternal salvation was in jeopardy.

Blame is a major staple of the Catholic psyche. The quickest and easiest route on the way to martyrdom is blame. There's always someone or something to blame. I can even blame myself for anything I want from being too stupid to being just generally not good enough.

So based on Dan's theory, my MS served me well. It was a condition from which I suffered, for which I sacrificed and meant I could view myself as a martyr.

Perfect.

I hadn't thought of Catholicism and multiple sclerosis existing hand-in-hand on the same path to my salvation but it made sense in a twisted kind of way. Now all I had to do was figure out how to be a whole and complete person without believing I had to suffer in order to validate my existence.

I was a good person. Why couldn't I be a whole and complete person and be happy and healthy at the same time?

Questioning

I was born and raised Catholic but I hadn't been a practicing Catholic since high school. Thinking about that, I realized I had asked a lot of questions about this religion when I was still in grade school and the answers I came to had a lingering effect into my adulthood.

For instance, praying. There was the rosary. I read a book in my late twenties called *The Yoga Aphorisms of Pantanjoli*. It was a comparison of Hinduism, Judaism and Catholicism. The author described the rosary as the Catholic version of a Hindu mantra. I liked that.

When I was in grade three I remember trying really hard to be seriously religious. At recess, I walked back and forth on the playground fingering the rosary in my pocket saying a prayer for each bead I held. I think I was expecting to be suddenly hit by a profound and overwhelming sense of spirit. Like the children at Fatima, I wanted to be struck by a powerful wave of discovery and knowledge that would leave me standing in the schoolyard hollering "Hallelujah" at the sky. But, it didn't happen.

I walked back and forth along the chain-link fence that separated the schoolyard and me from Lake St. Louis, the original polluted lake. It was spring and I thought that would be a good time to do my rosary practice. Spring meant Easter and we had just gotten over Lent. Spring also meant winter thaw. The problem was the chain-link fence. It might've separated me from the thawing lake but it didn't separate me from the sight and smell of dead fish rotting along the shoreline exposed by the melting ice. My commitment for saying the rosary didn't last long.

The prayers I really got a kick out of were the Indulgences. These are prayers designed to get you out of Purgatory faster. My first prayer book had a section just for the Prayers of Indulgence. Apparently, when you committed a sin it came with a sentence of time to spend in Purgatory for the transgression. I always wanted to see a list like a menu of how much time in Purgatory was required for each type of offence committed. I never saw a list like that any-where. For instance, what I wanted to know was if a lie was worth two days in Purgatory, how many days did you get for eating a hot dog on a Friday at a friend's birthday party? Those were two different issues as I saw it. In the case of telling a lie, you had a choice: You could tell the truth or you could lie. It was totally up to you. You knew if you told the truth you were okay. If you told a lie you knew that was wrong. It was a sin. It was a punishable offence and that meant time in Purgatory. But how much time? A day? A year?

See, when I was a kid, there was a rule about eating meat on Friday. Catholics didn't do it. In the case of a friend's birthday party, say it wasn't a fellow Catholic classmate but a neighbor friend from across the street, a Protestant friend. This could pose a serious dilemma. Say the birthday party for this Protestant neighbor friend was held on a Friday after school which included dinner. Your friend's mother had spent a large part of the day preparing for the party, putting up decorations and getting the food ready so every-body got fed.

Did you stand by the Catholic rules and turn down the hot dog offered at the birthday party, disappointing your friend's mother when all she was trying to be was a gracious hostess? Or did you accept the mustard-slathered dog on your Protestant friend's birthday and suffer the ecclesiastic consequences? Was God really watching this particular situation and keeping score on all those sinning eight-year-olds? Weren't there more important things for Him to be keeping track of like the Russians and the Americans building atomic bombs? I hoped He was watching those guys because we were already doing practice drills at school just in case there was an attack.

Was the Friday night Protestant birthday party the first test from God that a Catholic grade school child faced? Was a stint in Purgatory worth not insulting your friend's mother and not hurting your friend's feelings? Did good intentions mitigate the severity of the offense committed by accepting a hot dog at a birthday party on a Friday?

It was a birthday party. It was the celebration of a milestone in another human being's life, my neighbor, my friend. I always wanted to credit God with a little more compassion than blackening my soul with another stain and punishing me in Purgatory for committing the sin of being polite.

I think this was the kind of situation where I began to separate God from the church in my grade school mind. If He was all-knowing and all-loving as we were taught, certainly He would understand that our hearts were in the right place when we chose to eat a hot dog and make our friend and our friend's mother happy on a special occasion. Surely He wouldn't put a big "X" on my soul's scorecard for doing that. Surely, He had more important things to do than monitor hot dog consumption by Catholics around the world on a Friday night.

While time-for-crime lists weren't handy for reference, the Prayers of Indulgence did give me an exact day count for saying them. One prayer could get me three less days in Purgatory and another could get me ten. I used to look for the most time-effective prayers and say them one after the other. They didn't take long to say and if I got a couple of big ones said in a row, I could knock a month off Purgatory without too much effort. And then there was Confession. I could go to Confession, tell the priest my sins, say the prayers he assigned as my penance and wipe my soul clear so I could start all over again.

I wasn't particularly impressed by priests because I think I had a disconnect between the ones that stood at the front of the church behind the altar on Sunday and those I saw from a young age who were friends of my parents. These friends of my parents had grown up together, had gone to the same schools and knew each other's families. They had a lot of personal history in common. When these friends decided they had received a calling and entered religious life to become priests, that history wasn't lost.

When I met them, they were sitting in our backyard or another relative's yard at a barbecue. They wore trousers and short sleeve shirts and not the traditional floor length black cassocks with the hint of a white collar at the throat. They would be holding a beer and introduced to the neighbors simply by their first names. While we were told these men were priests, it was also made clear to us children that they were here at the barbecue off duty, so to speak. We were told they would be introduced by their first names to the neighbors so the neighbors wouldn't feel awkward about meeting a Catholic priest. They were family friends. As kids, we didn't know them as anything different than their first names either. So it's not that I didn't respect them as priests. I don't think I connected their religious calling with being anything other than family friends.

Having said all of that, I know people for whom the Catholic faith is a great comfort. They are devout Catholics and for them it all works. I had too many questions and I didn't get answers that satisfied me. When I had questions I was told I had to take it on faith that this was the way things were. I was sure God had a much better explanation. After all, He was God.

I'm still glad I had that Catholic upbringing. It gave me a set of values that I lean on and work from every day. For me, God will always be an old, white man with long white hair and a beard. At my most confused and angry about the MS, I called God every name in the book. Whenever I did that, really let Him have it, He always waited until I had finished my rant and then He would do something really nice for me. Sometimes it was a phone call from just the right person to talk to at that moment. Or I learned something about a situation I had been dreading that was completely different from the outcome I had braced for. I learned that when I yelled at God, He responded by doing something nice. I couldn't stay mad but when this horrendous medical insult that had been hurled at my life made holding a fork difficult and food landed in my lap, I felt completely justified hurling it right back at Him.

Martyr Heroine

Using how I quit smoking as the model for how to quit being addicted to feeling bad, I started to make progress slowly but surely. When I quit smoking it was suggested I figure out when I smoked, how many cigarettes a day I smoked, and why I picked up a cigarette at a particular time. When I realized I was repeatedly running an angry scenario in my mind with me as the victim of an undeserved injustice, even recognizing that my mind was running one of those non-stop victim scenarios was a major first step in being conscious that I was doing it at all. Only then could I make the effort to stop it.

Anything could set my mind off and running on an anger tangent: something that happened at work, rush-hour traffic, an unscheduled television show interrupting a program I wanted to see. The anger scenario was always somebody else's fault but I was always the one paying the consequences.

The instructions for quitting smoking said when I felt the urge to have a cigarette I should do something to distract myself until the urge passed. So that's what I did with the angry mind scenarios. Housework was a great distraction. Pulling out the vacuum, washing the kitchen floor or getting the laundry done were favourite activities. Not only did they change my focus, they also left me with a wonderful sense of accomplishment. With practice, I got faster at catching myself in mid-scenario and it got easier to tell myself to stop it by distracting my thoughts with another activity that filled the space in my head. I may not have been moving very well at this early stage of dealing with the MS but my apartment was looking pretty good.

What began to emerge for me was a fine distinction between victim and heroine. I started to realize I wasn't some overwhelmed weakling of a victim in my angry mind-movies. I was, in fact, a heroine. In the angry mind-movies I was the heroine who had been victimized. I was the martyr heroine. As a heroine, I was strong even though nasty life had overwhelmed me for an unguarded moment. When I imagined myself righting the wrong, I was powerful. Those unfortunates who experienced my self-righteous wrath, wilted at the awesome slash of my scathing remarks.

Take that, you lesser life forms. Yes. That felt good.

But before I could experience how good it felt to vanquish my "enemies", I had to feel bad. In this space between feeling bad followed by my imaginary struggle with the foe and my resulting triumph was where the addiction lived.

I started to use the drama of the strong but temporarily overpowered heroine to turn my addiction to feeling bad around. If I thought of myself as a victim I was weak, unsafe against the slightest of tissue breezes and trapped in a box I couldn't get out of. If I thought of myself as a heroine, I was strong and the box was no match for me. I was creating the angry scenarios in my mind; therefore, I was creating the box. If I created the box, I could also destroy it. If I was a victim, I was an overcooked noodle stuck in a box and nothing was ever going to change. So I chose to be the heroine and break out of that boxed-in mindset. I realized I was stronger than I gave myself credit for.

Thinking of me as a heroine instead of a victim shifted my view of myself and that was good. I became conscious of when I was running those anger movies in my head. The episodes happened less frequently but the feeling of being a martyr stuck. I may have been the heroine who broke down the box but I was still attached to feeling bad. How come I didn't lose that feeling? If the anger and my need for repeating the scenarios in my head were subsiding, why was I still feeling like a martyr?

Wherever the Information Comes From

Isn't it amazing how a word or two can make all the difference in how you understand an idea? I was beating all around the bush with words like Catholic and sacrifice, God, prayer, victim, etc. I was working diligently to become conscious of angry mind-movies, recognizing them and stopping the behaviour. And yet with all that work, I wondered why I had taken on this idea of being a breast-beating martyr and why I still felt, even with that description, I hadn't quite got it.

Then one day an audio tape caught my eye. It was a Lazaris tape and it was about self-pity.

That's it.

The two words that refined the space I had in my understanding of myself were self and pity. That hadn't occurred to me before. At this point in my learning evolution, I had come to understand that people and information crossed my path when I needed them and I was ready to hear what they had to say. I was now apparently confident enough to trust that process and recognized it when it was happening. Sometimes it was as obvious as a man I didn't know handing me a book and sometimes a scene in a movie could inspire an understanding. In this case, it was the title of an audiotape I saw out of the corner of my eye that snagged my attention and brought forward new thoughts. I had to pay attention. I bought the tape and when I listened to it, it rang more bells and whistles for me than a win at a slot machine. The information it contained was exactly what I needed at that moment, of course.

It was all about self-pity or self-importance as Lazaris called it. I identified with the 'struggler'. Lazaris' description of the struggler is someone who on the outside "…doesn't feel sorry for themselves on the surface; they're not bemoaning their fate; they're not critical; but they are struggling and they enjoy their struggle. They do 10 extra things, they work 5 times as hard, they re-do things 4 or 5 times. They struggle at getting their reality to work. They work harder than anybody. 'I'm not complaining. I just want you to know and I want you to appreciate all that I'm doing'."

Oh man, that's me.

When it came to his description of what the struggler personality was like on the inside he got even more accurate. His description of the rescuer/saviour said in part, "'Poor me. Look at how hard I have to work. Poor me. They never appreciate how wonderful I am. Poor me. I have to take time out from my life in order to save them'. Little realizing that those of you who are professional saviours - that *is* your life. You're not taking time out from it'."

This stuff is getting hard to hear.

But I kept listening because it was right on the money. I had never heard my problem articulated so clearly or more accurately and as much as I hated to admit it, I identified with every syllable.

Lazaris followed up his descriptions of self-pity with their ramifications. The ramification that reached out and spoke the loudest to me said that by practicing self-pity I would "end up feeling like a powerless child, a powerless child who projects Mother onto all women and Father onto all men, and resents the world and everybody in it. And that's why you feel like it's all right to manipulate through weakness. That's why you feel that it's all right to use your self-pity."

Manipulate through weakness – oh my God, I have MS. And I feel it's okay to use my self-pity? Am I doing that? I am doing that. Oh my God, I am doing that.

He had a plan for how to work with self-pity that included recognizing it. He said, "Acknowledge it for what it is – it's an illusionary game that you are choosing to play. You are not trapped in self-pity. You have put yourself there. You are not helplessly unable to get out of it. You have chosen quite calculatingly to put yourself into it."

That was a reassuring statement because it wiped out any leftover semblance of victim that might have been floating in the air around me. Finally, he had this amazing direction for me:

"If you want to get off self-pity, then it is a process of forgiving yourself by understanding where that self-pity began. For truly so, it did begin in your childhood. It was a survival mechanism to get you through tough times when you were too young to speak for yourself. It was a way of cocooning, of hiding out, until you were old enough, capable enough to fight off and defend yourself. It is a survival mechanism that is no longer productive. And you can forgive yourself for it. To change it, stop doing it. Understand the ramifications, what it looks like, what causes it, where its ramifications apply, acknowledge your payoffs and see the value of those payoffs reversed. Forgive yourself and then stop. Finally, release."

It was a survival mechanism begun in childhood that was no longer productive. But it didn't stop there. It was attached to another feeling, feeling I was not good enough.

Do I ever get to the bottom of this? Where does it end?

Île d'Orléans

There is an island in the St. Lawrence River directly across from Québec City called Île d'Orléans, the Isle of Orleans. Québec City was founded in 1608 by the explorer Samuel de Champlain. In 1659, Île d'Orléans was the site of the first land grants given out in Canada then known as the French colony of New France. There were fifty-three land grants given out and my family got three of them. The three parcels of land went to Jacques Asseline, his brother David and their cousin René.

My father was made aware of a book entitled *Les Asselin* when his cousin, who still lived in Montréal, called to tell him about it. My father's cousin had been contacted by a woman named Jacqueline Faucher Asselin from Québec City to get information about our branch of the family. She had written the book inspired by her children's homework assignment to trace the family tree. She went beyond the project and seven years after she started researching the family genealogy, her book was published. At the time of publication, there were still sections of the family tree that Jacqueline hadn't been able to tie into one of the main three lines of descendents from

128

Jacques, David or René. Our family was in one of those incomplete sections. My father ordered one copy of the book for the family and I ordered one copy of the book just for me.

After our copies of the book arrived we read them avidly. My great-great-grandfather was a man whose first name was Élie, not a very common name. I read through the entire book and found only eleven references to men named Élie. What I found particularly interesting looking through the Asselin book was how the first names followed each other from one generation to the next. They were like stepping stones. People were always named after someone in the family – a parent, a grandparent, an aunt, an uncle, a cousin. I then tried to match up the dates for births, deaths, and marriages to figure out where my great-great-grandfather Élie would connect us with one of the three original Asselins.

I figured out that we probably connected with Jacques' descendents. My father went to the provincial museum and got a copy of the 1888 Census of Canada to prove my theory and found the names we were looking for. We sent all the information we had gathered to Jacqueline. She wrote back that because of our amateur detective work she had not only been able to connect our family group to Jacques' family tree but she had also been able to make the connection for four other family groups. Our branch of the family was now officially designated J11 which means I am a direct descendent of Jacques and an eleventh generation Canadian. So in May, 1998 when a friend invited me to come to Québec City for a visit, at the top of my list of things to do was go to Île d'Orléans.

The Anglophone and the Separatist

I met the friend who invited me to Québec City years before in Jasper. She had enrolled at the University of Laval to participate in a French immersion course for a year. By the time spring came around, she was homesick for a familiar face and since I wasn't married or caught up with raising children, I could easily accept her invitation to get on a plane and go for a visit.

Île d'Orléans is only a fifteen minute drive out of Québec City across a bridge onto the island. We stopped at the information building we saw as soon as we came off the bridge. The woman at the counter told us that as time went on and the population of the island increased, the succeeding generations moved a little farther along and built the next parish. Hence there were six parishes on the island. The first and oldest parish was Ste. Famille. She had a list of which families belonged to each parish and as Jacques was one of the original settlers, Ste. Famille is the church he belonged to along with his brother and cousin. We were told there was a monument on the property that Jacques had owned. The church, the monument and the property were just a little way down the road from the information building. We would find it easily.

We drove past the church and almost immediately saw a large three-sided rock near the road on a piece of property with a small white house. On each side of the rock was a name – one side was Jacques, another side was David and the third side was René. The last name on each side was a different spelling variation of the name Asselin. Probably Jacques, David and René were illiterate. At that time only the clergy or the wealthy would have been educated. The illiterate person would have been dependent on somebody else to record their names on official documents so the spelling could change depending on who did the writing.

My friend took a couple of pictures of me standing with my cane beside the side of the rock showing Jacques' name. When we were done looking at the property, we drove back down the road to the church of Ste. Famille and went around it down the hill to the cemetery where we parked the car. I was interested to see what names were on the headstones and how far back the dates on the headstones went. I got out of the car and leaned up against the open door with my cane. I was strong enough to stand there but certainly not strong enough to walk around the graveyard. My friend took on that job and shouted back the Asselin name on a headstone from time to time and the date that was on it. The oldest date we found for someone named Asselin was 1845. Between 1659 and 1845 a lot of changes had obviously occurred. The woman at the information building told us the church itself had been rebuilt three times since first constructed. In the graveyard, no physical evidence remained of who had been buried there prior to 1845.

A man and a teenage girl were sitting on the church steps eating lunch out of paper bags while we were scouting the cemetery. They heard us shouting back and forth and knew that we spoke English, so when the man came down to the graveyard from the church he asked in English with a French accent, "Who are you looking for?" I answered in what I hoped was correct French, "Mon ancestre Jacques Asselin." "Jacques Asselin?" he answered practically shouting. "I'm looking for my ancestor—" and he said his ancestor's name. I smiled and nodded and when he realized the name meant nothing to me, he said, "Wait. I have a book." Off he went excitedly to the parking lot to retrieve a book from his car.

`He came back holding a soft cover book that was thinner than the Asselin genealogy. He showed me the cover and pointed to the last name. "That's me," he said. "That's my last name and that's my ancestor." It still didn't mean anything to me. "He knew Jacques Asselin. They were friends. They bought the land together." He flipped open the book and found the page that had the map of Île d'Orléans showing the parcels of land that were given out in the 1659 land grants and the names of the owners. We had exactly the same map in the book *Les Asselin*.

His book told the story of how his ancestor came to New France in 1652. He was indentured as a servant to a former governor of Québec. He remained his servant for six years. In 1658, when his brother arrived in New France, the brother leased a piece of land from the parish of Ste. Famille on Île d'Orléans. The following year his ancestor and "an associate, Jacque[s] Asseline" purchased most of the land his ancestor's brother had leased the previous year. The purchase price was three hundred French pounds. Somewhere along the line this man's ancestor and mine knew each other and pooled their resources to purchase property in the new world. More than three centuries later, on a beautiful, warm Tuesday afternoon in May, the direct descendents of those two pioneers, partners, and neighbours stood in the graveyard of the church where their ancestors' bones had long since turned to dust and shared their stories.

He earned his living writing. So did I. I was born in Montréal and lived there till I was fifteen. He lived in Montréal with his wife and two teenage daughters. He introduced us to his older daughter who we had seen eating lunch with him on the church steps. His younger daughter was in the car. She was apparently unhappy about something and had decided to stay there. MS was something else we had in common. He said he noticed my cane and how I was moving and he asked me if I had multiple sclerosis. I said yes and he said he thought that's what the problem was from the way I moved. He said he was being tested for MS, too. He said he wanted to come to Île d'Orléans to see where his family history started and share the experience with his daughters in case he waited too long and wouldn't be able to drive from Montréal to Québec City later. He jokingly suggested that perhaps the doctors would discover that multiple sclerosis also started on Île d'Orléans.

As our conversation was coming to an end, he said to me, "So, you were born in Montréal and you lived there and your last name is Asselin but you don't speak French?" I smiled, shrugged my shoulders and said "Anglophone." He took a step to walk away and then stopped. Indicating himself with a hand tap to his chest he said, "Je suis maudit séparatiste." His declaration caught me so off guard I burst out laughing. He walked away waving his hand goodbye over his shoulder.

When my friend and I returned to her car, she said she was shocked that I laughed after he called himself a separatist and wanted to know why I had reacted that way. I told her I took his remark as a back-handed compliment. He had done a play on words. The more familiar expression in Québec was 'maudit Anglais' and it was quite derogatory. That's what I was – English, English with a French last name who only spoke English. That kind of person was not welcome in Québec. He called himself a 'maudit séparatiste' acknowledging who each of us was and the fact that we had spent over an hour talking about all the things we have in common and we had enjoyed meeting.

Three-hundred-plus years after the fact, two complete strangers meet in a graveyard on Île d'Orléans in the middle of the St. Lawrence River. We are both direct descendents of our respective family trees. Our ancestors were friends who crossed the Atlantic Ocean from Normandy, France six years apart in the mid 1600's. They pooled their resources, bought two strips of land beside each other on the island and invested everything they had in this new world. In addition to ancestry, the two strangers both write for a living and have MS. He has come from Montréal and I have come from Edmonton but on this lovely afternoon in May, we are both here. Once again, the Universe has arranged things just so.

Grocery Shopping
in Bridgewater

Grocery shopping in Bridgewater, Nova Scotia opened up a whole new world for me. I was losing a little more balance every time I went out and I bent over the cane in order to keep what balance I had. My internal organs felt scrunched and I longed to be able to stand up straight and not feel like I was going to fall down. I was standing with my cane in the driveway at my friends' house and fell straight backwards after I threw my head back laughing at something funny somebody said. Not so funny.

We had to go for groceries so I offered to push the shopping cart while the others picked items off the shelves. I put my cane in the basket and discovered something fabulous – when I was pushing the shopping cart I had something to hang on to for balance and at the same time I was walking straight up. My posture was wonderful, my internal organs were relieved and I felt secure. I came home from Nova Scotia excited about my discovery. I could get rid of the cane. All I needed was a shopping cart to get around.

Could I get a shopping cart in my car?

I was describing all of this in a session with Dan and talking about what a relief it was to stand up straight and move without being worried about losing my balance. We pitched ideas back and forth and came up with using something like cross country ski poles to walk with. That type of ski pole is longer than downhill ski poles which meant I could stand up straight, stay balanced, and walk while alternating which pole was planted and which pole was swinging forward to take the next step.

I was thoroughly excited by our brainstorming session. When I came home I immediately started to phone sporting goods stores to get prices on cross-country ski poles. I wasn't worried about the pointy ends on the poles. In winter, they would be handy cutting into snow and ice. As for the other seasons or walking on flooring surfaces, I would figure out how to handle them.

After dinner the condo buzzer rang. It was Dan. His arrival was totally unexpected. When I opened the door he was standing there holding tall poles in his hand. I took them immediately out of his grasp and started walking across the living room rug alternating the poles with each step. He explained he had made them himself from copper piping he had found in the alley near his home some time ago. The piping was probably leftovers from a plumbing job he figured that was being thrown away. He brought the copper pipe home thinking one day it might come in handy for something. Little did he know he would be making walking poles out of them for me.

After our session in his office earlier that day, he went home and cut the thin copper pipes for height and went to a sporting goods store where he found a pair of children's ski poles. He used the hand grips from the children's poles for the top of the copper pipes and on the bottom of the pipes he put small plastic footings he got from something else he had. He could see the poles were a bit too long for me as I went back and forth across the living room but he said he could cut a couple of inches off the bottom and make them a better height for me.

I was stunned. My appointment with Dan had been just before noon hour and now, seven hours later, he stood at my front door with copper walking poles he had made for me complete with hand grips and plastic footings. I was so excited.

Oh my God, he heard me.

Not only had he heard me, he acted on what I was imagining out loud and created it. What was so surprising to me was that it was a man who had listened and a man who had made those ideas reality for me. I don't remember that happening with a man before, a man listening, hearing and acting on something I said, something I needed. Then again maybe I had only asked for what I needed before in a whisper, if at all.

The next morning, my father brought a walker home for me to try from a medical supply store. It was a good walker but I still had to lean forward to use it and couldn't stand straight up while walking. The poles had another advantage over the walker. When I came to stairs with the walker I would be stopped whereas I could go up and down stairs with the walking poles, one step at a time.

My father and I did a bit more fine tuning of the walking poles by getting proper rubber grips on the bottom ends. We purchased picks that clamped onto the bottom of the poles. In winter, I could flip the picks down to walk on snow and ice. In the summer or on floors, I would flip the picks up out of the way in favour of the rubber footings for balance.

The walking poles became a huge part of my life for the next three years and I kept them even after I had to start using a wheelchair. I believe there will be a day when I use them again. Whether I do or not, I will always have them because of what they mean to me. I was heard by a man who thought my idea was valid. But what they really represented to me in that moment was *I am valid*. Those poles are in my closet now. That's okay. I know where they are.

Thank you, Dan.

Being Good Enough

Another Lazaris tape that came across my path discussed what it was to be good enough. I wallowed in self-pity so it followed that I believed I wasn't good enough. I believed I didn't deserve good things. Other people could have wonderful things happen to them. That was fine but good things certainly didn't come in my direction. I wasn't good enough to deserve them. That's what I believed.

Obviously, good things did happen for me but it seemed like I just fell into them. They were some kind of happenstance or fluke. They weren't necessarily mistakes but I always thought sooner or later the gods would discover they had bestowed their gifts on a lesser life form that was flawed, defective and plain not good enough to have them. Sooner or later "they" were going to figure that out. Maybe I wasn't grateful enough for the good things that did come my way to keep the momentum going. I think I believed that a certain amount of good things were all right but too many good things weren't acceptable. The extras should be pushed away in order to stay humble. There was also a qualitative level of good things. For instance, a good thing that was 'all right' or 'okay' was acceptable to aspire to.

A good thing that was 'fabulous' was right out of my league. Maybe that was part of my Catholic learning.

I believed I shouldn't be so audacious as to imagine I had dreams that could be pursued by doing the activities necessary to turn those dreams into reality. I had absolutely no concept of what it was to create a five-year plan for myself. I could not conceive of creating a list of goals and an action plan to accomplish them. I applied that belief across the board – dreams, relationships, money – whatever it was, I would have just enough of it to get by and then it would either stop in its tracks or completely fall apart. It's what I expected so my negative beliefs became self-fulfilling prophecies.

I didn't recognize what a struggle it was always acting like I was working towards good things, that good things were coming my way, when in my heart of hearts, I didn't believe it. It was a completely unnecessary stress I imposed on myself

Where did I get it into my head that I wasn't good enough? Why didn't I think I could have a great relationship, marriage and children, own a house, have enough money to afford whatever other good things normal people dream about and accomplish?

How come I didn't think that way? What would life be like if I could turn that belief around? What if I truly did believe that I was good enough? What would happen then? What would life be like if I truly did believe I deserved good things? Even thinking those questions caused my stomach to tighten up as if I had been caught thinking things that were prohibited. Thinking the way I did certainly wasn't getting me anywhere. I was stuck. My thinking was going to have to change if I was going to move forward in any direction but I didn't have a clue how I was going to do that.

My belief about being not good enough was so deep-rooted. Where did it come from?

Lazaris suggested it could have been something I was taught or conditioned to believe by a well-meaning parent or grandparent. Maybe I had somehow failed an unspoken demand for perfection in expectations of terrific grades at school. Maybe now, thirty to forty years later I don't think I deserve because I failed to meet those expectations. Even if something like that was the reason why I felt the way I did, why would I have taken such a misunderstanding so ferociously to heart for so long?

Or maybe I just assumed it.

Sigh...

The Swan Dive

My brother was born in the middle of October, which meant when he was able to join us at the community outdoor pool for his first summer he would have been eight months old. For that summer and for the summers that followed I remember him sitting patiently at the side of the pool while my parents, my sister and I took turns swimming and minding him. He must've felt he was getting enough time in the pool because I never remember him being fussy or whining or demanding time in the water. He watched everybody else playing and swimming and diving off the board until it was his turn to be taken into the water again. I also never remember anybody trying to get him to swim. We would hold him in our arms and swish him from side to side in the water or bounce on our feet up and down getting him wet and cooled off in the hot and humid Montréal summers.

Then one day, the summer he was four years old turning five in the fall, I remember hearing the lifeguard shout, "Cathy. Your brother's on the diving board." I was in the pool in the shallow end. I turned to look at the deep end and there was my brother standing at the end of the diving board. My father was also in the pool almost at the deep end and he turned to see my brother standing on the diving board as well. Before anyone could react, my brother bounced on the end of the board sending him up in the air. He bent over and touched his toes before he slipped into the water in a perfect straight-line. It was the most beautiful, simple, effortless swan dive anyone had ever seen a four-year-old do.

I was so stunned to see my brother standing on the diving board, never mind see him do his perfect swan dive, that it took a moment before I realized he had gone into the deep end and he didn't know how to swim. I saw my father. If anything was wrong he could've gotten to my brother in a heartbeat but he didn't move. I remember seeing the lifeguard half standing out of his chair watching the deep end intently but not moving a muscle. Everyone and everything had stopped and was focused on the surface of the water at the deep end of the pool.

In a matter of seconds, my brother popped to the surface like a baby sea otter. He immediately flipped over onto his back, waving his arms at his side and kicking his legs, he splashed across the water to the ladder at the side of the pool and climbed out. He started to walk back towards the diving board. The lifeguard shouted at him to stop. Apparently, four-year-old kids who didn't know how to swim couldn't just go bouncing off the diving board into the deep end like that. My father said it was okay, that he was there and would catch him if he needed help. So my brother did it again. He climbed onto the diving board, walked to the end, bounced up into the air, bent to touch his toes, and straightened his legs behind him as he slipped into the water. A moment later he popped to the surface, flipped over on his back, waving his arms and kicking his legs to propel him over to the ladder and he climbed out of the pool. No big deal. After that day he was allowed to dive to his heart's content between 5 p.m. and 6 p.m. on Saturdays when the swimming crowd had begun to thin out to go home for dinner.

I've thought about that a fair amount since being in the wheel-chair. My little brother sat on the sidelines at a community pool for four summers going on five and watched his way to a perfect swan dive. He actually made a choice by doing that. He could've done a cannonball off the diving board like so many kids and adults he had watched. He could have done what other little kids did when they learn to dive, standing at the edge of the pool, hands clasped over his head, bent over creating the intention of diving and then just jumped into the pool anyway. But he didn't do that. He chose to do a swan dive off the diving board into the deep end of the pool.

There were a number of people at the free swim Saturday and Sunday afternoons who did swan dives off our little one metre board so he did have numerous occasions to watch them do it. But it fas-cinates me that his young brain saw something he liked and had the discretion to choose what it was he would do the first time he got on the board and it wasn't a cannonball. Maybe he liked how controlled the dive looked. A person walks to the end of the board and when he gets there he makes a little bounce with his step raising one knee so he goes down on the board harder and creates a larger bounce that seems to push him up into the air. And then almost leisurely in midair he bends at the waist, touches his toes and his legs swing up behind him before his hands and head slip into the water, his pointed toes following behind.

What was it that made my brother get up and walk over to the diving board that day? How did he know he could do that dive? How did he know he would come to the surface? Did he understand it was the deep end of the pool? Did he just assume he would because he'd seen other people go below the surface and come up again? And when he came to the surface how did he know what to do to get from the middle of the deep end to the side of the pool so he could climb up the ladder and get out? How did he know that by waving his arms and kicking his legs he could travel across the water? Did he know just because he'd seen other people do that?

All he did for four summers going on five was observe, and imagine to the point where his body believed it could do that and it did.

By watching and imagining, the neural pathways in his brain were wired and connected to the muscles in his body in a way he would need to accomplish that swan dive. And then one day he walked onto the diving board, bounced into the air with a knowledge so absolute about what he was going to do, it stunned the rest of us. But for him it was as natural as breathing. He just did it.

If I imagine buttoning a shirt, buttering my toast, or writing my name, would the tremors in my arms and the weakness in my hands disappear? If I watch and observe and imagine will I create new neural pathways that will allow me to stand? Christopher Reeve worked very hard with doctors and therapists and specialists for nine years because he believed he could walk again. When all was said and done he didn't walk but what he did do was move his baby finger, voluntarily. He wasn't supposed to be able to do that but he did. My then four-year-old brother wasn't supposed to be able to do a swan dive but he did. We just don't understand how it all works.

Thank goodness faith isn't dependent on intellect.

Dreaming is freeing.

Believing is empowering.

The How is just nuts and bolts.

Segment 7 – Change Involves

Change involves the deepest sort of self-doubt.
While struggling through change, the Pathfinder is between two selves:
his or her former identity is at least partially cracked
and a raw and fragile new carapace is trying to form
in the chilly air of uncertainty.

Gail Sheehy
Passages

Fix It

Healing is uneven, confusing, and mystifying work. Since the Second World War and the availability of antibiotics, we've come to think of healing as a straight line: we're sick; we go to the doctor; the doctor gives us a prescription for antibiotics and we get better. Done deal.

It became apparent to me that I didn't get into this predicament in a straight line, so there was no reason to think I could get out of it in a straight line either. The way out may not be straight, but the twists and turns of "the scenic route" offered views and points of interest I wouldn't have found otherwise.

Personal crises are double-edged swords. In my case, one edge of the sword made me lash out at anything or anyone who made me feel unsafe at this time of tremendous personal vulnerability. The other edge of the sword gave me time and space, more time and space than I would have given myself if I'd been left on my own to continue going down the path I was on. My diagnosis of MS not only scared me, it scared the people around me, too. Thank God family and friends didn't back off despite my hissing and spitting.

Healing, I was discovering, takes effort, imagination, and courage. There's nothing like a good dose of fear and panic to make you open to suggestion but it took me awhile – quite awhile – before I saw my condition as an opportunity. I could reach out now and choose the people and activities that would encourage and support me instead of giving my time and energy to those situations that drained me. The MS gave me permission to try new things.

I started to give myself permission to live my life. It turns out that's what I was healing. I was giving me permission to be who I was. For some reason, up to the moment I was diagnosed, I hadn't believed I deserved the time, the space, and the support I needed to go out and live my own life. What did I like? What did I enjoy? What did I know I could do? Why did I think I had to get permission from somewhere or someone else? Why did it never dawn on me I was the only one who could give me permission? That's what I was healing – giving myself permission to live as me. It turns out the MS was a symptom of my confused and twisted belief system.

The people and the information I needed were there. A lot of it had been there for a long time, sitting on my bookshelf or dormant in a memory bank. I started to realize that when I said "help", or "I can't", or "show me" something would happen. The phone rang with a caller I would never have expected or a complete stranger helped me in a store or the perfect parking space appeared. Something would change. Something I wouldn't have anticipated. What I needed to do was pay attention.

The healing process is messy but tomorrow, I learned, is always another day. My double-edged sword was both a burden and my shield. It was a struggle and my gift. Multiple sclerosis was my teacher, tough though it may be.

A New Day, New Cells

Today I gave birth to a new generation of cells. They say every twenty-four hours the body re-creates itself by shedding old cells and making new ones. When I stopped smoking I started creating new cells without nicotine. When I stopped playing the feel-bad-mind-movies I started to create cells without self-pity. Without self-pity I gave myself the gifts of possibility, forward momentum and opportunity. When I finally got some of my twisted emotional bad habits untangled, what did I see? I saw life without the Martyr Heroine.

What a relief.

And forward momentum brings (drum roll) –

Life in a wheelchair. (Cymbal crash)

Now there's a bombshell I didn't see coming.

I think the Martyr Heroine grew from a combination of two things. One was a misunderstanding and the other was a mistaken assumption. Both began in childhood and they created the basis for the toxic broth I called the Martyr Heroine.

The misunderstanding was my grandfather's death. When I tried to say Grandpa it came out Ganga so that's what stuck. Ganga died a week before I turned three. All of my earliest memories are of him – being in Val Morin at the country house my grandparents rented in summer; him picking up beetles from under the front door's wooden step and putting them in my pink plastic pail; being held by him walking into the lake until the water was up to his waist and tickling my toes; laughing and singing until we were red in the face and gasping for breath.

Back at home, he used to come over to our place pretty regularly on Sunday afternoons I was told. Apparently a little while after his funeral I said to my mother as a statement of fact, "Ganga's not coming anymore". She said no and that was all I was told. No one made an attempt to explain what happened. There were no stories about angels coming to take him to heaven. One minute he was there. The next minute he had a massive heart attack on a Saturday morning before going to work and now he was gone. Years later when I asked my mother about it, she said no one thought to explain it to a three-year-old because they would have thought I was too young to understand. I may not have had the vocabulary to include the word 'death' but I understood enough about the concept of 'going away' to make the statement to my mother that he wouldn't be coming over anymore.

Like little kids do, I figured it was something I did. I was responsible for the fact that he wasn't coming over anymore. I assumed it was my fault. A man I adored had left suddenly and without explanation and it was probably my fault. I didn't know what I had done but I probably did it. How often did that get played out in my relationships when I got older? If I cared for a man, I expected him to leave and most of the time he did. But if he hung around, then I left. And I think that behaviour might have gone back to that day in January, 1956 when my grandfather's heart attack meant he wouldn't be coming over anymore. The message my three year old brain got was that if I loved a man, he probably wouldn't stick around to be with me.

When my grandfather died I don't remember crying or acting any differently on the outside. Whatever confusion and upset I felt was probably bottled up on the inside. Then it started to fester.

The assumption I made in my childhood had to do with how I thought it was my job to make sure my mother was happy, my father was in a good mood, and I maintained the peace between me and my younger sister. One of the ways I could make my mother and father happy was not to cause them any problems at home and to be a terrific student. I remember being particularly worried about a math test I had in grade four. When I got 98/100 I was thrilled. I showed the test paper to my father with the teacher's handwriting in red ink across the top of the page -- 98/100. I was so relieved and so proud. He looked at the paper and said *"Ninety-eight?* What happened to the other two points?"

He was teasing but I didn't understand his sense of humor. I never forgot that. I guess everybody can tell a story about when they got shot down by someone they wanted to please. When you're young and emotionally dependent on a parent, it's hard to walk away from something like that and not feel the failure. Somewhere along the line, I made the decision to be responsible for other people's happiness at the expense of my own and that got bottled up inside as well.

I created my self-pity and stayed with it because it was a successful coping mechanism. I could keep what I really felt inside and not make a mess on the outside. But that was when I was a child. Now that I was seriously considering giving up the self pity, it was scary. I didn't know what life would be like without it. It could be worse. If I decided to be emotionally responsible for myself, I might experience another kind of pain, maybe more pain, says the child's belief system. Besides, how could I be so selfish and give up being emotionally responsible for others? How would they cope without me?

When the fear took over, I backed off being emotionally responsible for myself so I wouldn't experience the anticipated pain. The MS kicked in, my legs cratered, and I flipped into a manipulation mechanism to get others to look after *me*. I was living with my parents, Dan patiently listened to me wailing and wringing my hands, and Kevin carried me up the stairs from his office to my car. Once again, I was saved from being emotionally responsible for myself and safe from feeling overwhelming pain.

I became more aware of how these ideas got twisted and operated in me. If I sloughed off a set of old cells every day and created a batch of new ones then I should be able to put new ideas into the new cells and with conscious and consistent effort, be a brand-new person at the end of the day. I could be a brand-new person who got up the stairs from Kevin's office to my car on my own two feet.

The FDR Illusion

It was about the time I started using the walking poles that I saw a documentary on television about Franklin Roosevelt. A large part of the film focused on his polio. As I watched the program I was fascinated to see how he created the illusion of wellness that everyone around him bought into.

In the summer of 1921 while he was vacationing on Campobello Island in New Brunswick, he contracted polio. He was thirty-nine years old. In 1932, eleven years *after* being paralyzed, he was elected President of the United States.

Roosevelt was innovative in how he dealt with his paralysis. He swam to try to regain the strength in his legs. He discovered the benefits of bathing in the warm waters of mineral springs. He designed leg braces for himself so he could stand. As I recall, the program said the braces were made of iron. Roosevelt not only figured out how he could stand but also how he could appear to be walking with the help of his son. The iron braces were out of sight under Roosevelt's trousers. Father and son were the same height and his son supported his father standing in such a way that they were upright but appeared not to be leaning on each other for support as they took slow steps. Roosevelt kept his head tilted back slightly, wearing his hat at a bit of an angle. He smiled broadly like he had just heard a good joke. The two men walked arm-in-arm as if they had all the time in the world to enjoy a leisurely stroll on a pleasant afternoon. Roosevelt's son must have been incredibly strong to support his father wearing iron leg braces and make it look so casual and easy.

Roosevelt often rode in open convertibles so when the car was stopped he could reach out to people and talk to them without obstruction. His head and hat were tilted back just enough to give him a jaunty air and he had that smile on his face. Even when he had a cigarette holder clenched between his teeth he was smiling. My mother said she remembers seeing Roosevelt in newsreel film after he had finished giving a speech, reaching back to each one of his knees, hitting something on the braces underneath the trousers so his knees bent and he could sit down. That was normal. No one questioned it.

When he wasn't in public he used a wheelchair. The documentary cited an instance when Roosevelt fell out of his wheelchair at a White House dinner. One of the waiters simply picked him up, got him back in the chair and carried on with his serving duties. Roosevelt continued the conversation he was having and the press never reported the mishap.

It was as if the press and the public had agreed to participate in Roosevelt's illusion that he was just fine and everyone felt better for joining in the conspiracy. Everybody knew he had polio but no one made an issue of it. Nor did they seem to spend any time considering how remarkable it was that this man who suffered from a crippling illness was not only out and about living his life but he was doing it on a level that was extraordinary. His smile and optimistic nature, his creativity for problem-solving, his determination and strong, confident voice took the United States and most of the world through the Depression, World War II, three full terms and into his fourth term as President before his death in 1945. He created function and productivity for himself in a world that really wasn't prepared to credit someone with a disability. Even though nobody said anything about it specifically, I think people understood what he was doing subconsciously. Watching him, perhaps they felt if he can do it, so can I. Maybe that's how people weathered the economic and political storms of those decades.

The documentary inspired me. I'm an optimist by nature so I thought I should start using that part of my personality. I needed my family and my friends. I needed their energy and their love. I wanted them to be rooting for me. I needed them to allow me to be part of their lives. Feeling fearful, angry and frustrated didn't mean I had to show everybody how miserable I felt sometimes. I know I hated it when someone looked at me with pity and doleful eyes. Did I expect everyone to have infinite patience and sympathy for me when all I gave them was a continued display of pathetic gloom? That wasn't going to get me a lot of invitations.

I wanted to create the image that everything was fine with me, too. I wanted to give everybody around me the confidence that I was okay. If I got others to believe that then I could use their positive feedback to energize the efforts I had to make to live up to that image. I believed I was still useful and interesting and I wanted them to think that way about me, too. I needed others' support to help me give life a good shot.

It wasn't quite that easy because the effects of the MS were so variable for me at that point. I could feel physically different from one minute to the next. It was frustrating but I began to learn that if I felt crummy one minute, I would feel better in the next. There wasn't any rhyme or reason to it as far as I could tell. I started to trust that if I didn't feel well that feeling wasn't going to last forever. It would pass and probably pretty soon. When I felt better I tried to do more. If I started to feel lousy, I backed off for a while. Soon I would feel better. The good moments came around and I watched for them so

I could make progress. I paid less and less attention to the fatigue knowing it was temporary, too.

Thanks, Mr. Roosevelt.

"Let me get that for you."

When I first started to use the walking poles I was initially concerned about how I would handle opening a door. Both of my hands were occupied holding a pole and if I wanted to keep my balance I better keep holding onto them. But from the first outing, doors got opened for me. Men appeared out of nowhere and said "Let me get that for you." They would open the door and I would smile and say something silly like "I'll try to get there before your next birthday." Usually that got a laugh. The fact that I had accepted their offer of help to open a door, had a smile on my face, a normal speaking voice and a sense of humor was, I think, a great source of relief for the gentlemen. They were so pleasant and willing to help that I began to form a theory.

I think the walking poles gave men the opportunity and the confidence to be chivalrous. I began to think that men are naturally inclined to be helpful. They are problem solvers. When they saw me heading for a door, walking awkwardly, balanced by a pole in each hand, they saw it as their moment. The fact that I had a smile on my face signaled that if they offered help I probably wasn't going to yell at them in a feminist I-can-do-it-myself rant and shoot them down for their kind offer of assistance. They could be helpful, show their good manners, and live to tell the tale. Thank goodness for the women's movement but I began to think it had kicked the daylights out of men's confidence to be gallant and open a door for a lady.

Sometimes they would ask me what happened. A man would see me struggling along and assume I had sustained some kind of an injury. They would immediately launch into the story of how they could relate because of knee replacement surgery they had had or a broken leg they had suffered on a ski slope. I also discovered men are suckers for a southern accent. Sometimes when they asked what happened I would answer in a southern drawl that it had been a dance floor incident I'd rather not talk about. That would make them laugh, too. People were open to me when I used the walking poles but then I was open to receiving what they had to offer – their help.

As a matter of fact, those poles were quite the man-magnets. One of my friends used to say if you want to meet men just go out with Cathy. Stand her on a corner with those poles and then take your pick. She dropped me off one day in front of a building and there was no one around. I stood on the sidewalk while she quickly turned the car around and parked in the designated handicapped stall in front of the building. By the time she got out of the car and walked up to where she had left me, I was at the front door of the building with three young guys who were holding the doors open for me. After we were inside the building and out of earshot of those nice young men, she turned to me and shouted, "How do you do that?"

Now, the wheelchair comes with another set of reactions from people but to the best of my ability at any given moment in time, the smile is on my face, my voice is clear and with maybe some kind of a smart Alec remark. A sense of humour makes up for a lot of ground when you need to be pushed.

The Patio

I was sitting on the front patio of the co-op I live in with a neigh-bour who was also in a wheelchair. We were admiring the flowers in the garden, enjoying the beautiful summer day. My neighbour commented to me that she thought people's attitudes were getting better when they saw someone in a wheelchair. Polio was her story for being in a chair. She said when she was younger people would see her in the chair and assume that she was probably – you know – not very intelligent, retarded they used to call it, she explained. But she thought that had changed. She wanted to know if I had ever experienced that attitude from people.

Not that so much I said. What I had noticed was that when people saw me in the wheelchair sometimes they assumed there must be something *else* wrong with me. Apparently I couldn't walk but there could also be something else wrong. I told her about the time I was in the grocery store and a nice lady put her hand on my arm, leaned down so we were face to face and then said loudly with crisp annunciation –

Have you been en-joy-ing the love-ly weath-er we're hav-ing?

It's Genetic

I came back from my trip to Île d'Orléans declaring to Dan, "It's genetic." I had stood on the property owned by my ancestor. I had stood in the graveyard of the first parish and met a man whose ancestor was the partner and neighbor of mine. I had MS and he was being tested to see if he had it. He said we were going to find out that MS started on Île d'Orléans and we had laughed. Do I really think Île d'Orléans is where MS started? No. But there was something in what he said that made me think.

I'm an eleventh generation Canadian. The Mayflower only beat my people to North America by thirty-nine years. In my family's genealogy book there is a picture of the baptismal font in the church in the town of Bracquemont, Normandy where my ancestor, Jacques, was baptized. The Catholicism in our family went back that far and further. It was documented. Over three hundred years of knowing we had come into this life flawed with Original Sin. Over three hundred years of knowing we weren't good enough. If we practiced our religion faithfully, stayed away from sin, and confessed when we didn't, we had a shot at heaven.

Maybe being taught that I was doomed by sin before I took my first breath and believing I wasn't good enough, set me up to host an illness like MS. Maybe it's the kind of illness that feeds on negative thinking. Maybe being born Catholic didn't cause the illness but that religion's belief system gave it a fertile place to develop. It could be that the nature of an illness like MS isn't just the physicality of the ailment like catching the flu bug. Maybe after believing generation after generation that we are flawed, inadequate, and not good enough, those thoughts creep into our bones and seep into our cells – physically, mentally, spiritually – a body incorporates the negative. And then maybe something happens, the negative belief system gets set off somehow and before you know it there's a flunky in a neurologist's office handing you a card with a number to call when you want to get your wheelchair.

It's genetic. It's been over three hundred documented years. After that much time believing you're not good enough, it's more than negative thinking. It's cellular.

Okay. Now what? I know it's there. I've recognized it. When it's in my cells, how do I get rid of it?

I don't remember what Dan's answer was. It was probably something sage like – could be. I had quit smoking, remember? I was applying those same Canadian Lung Association how-to-quit suggestions to how to turn my thinking around but this was genetic. This was really deep. I could probably start with those suggestions but I was really going to have to think about this one.

What do you do to get rid of a belief system you're carrying when you and your people have been carrying it so long it's deeper than a plantar wart? When I was a kid I had a plantar wart burned out one time. How do you burn out a belief system that reaches back eleven generations?

The Point of No Return

My father was a moody man. When he was up and things were going his way he was terrific. He loved comedians. As a kid, I remember him laughing so hard at Jonathan Winters and Red Skelton he could barely breathe. In later years, the Royal Canadian Air Farce and Bill Mahr could put him away. I remember him laughing more when I was younger than what I saw when I was living with my parents after we moved into the condo together. Maybe it was the stress and strain of three adults living together and one of them, the adult child, not coping very gracefully with the variable and apparently progressive MS.

My diagnosis was primary progressive multiple sclerosis. That meant I was going to hell in a hand basket, do not pass Go, do not collect $200, there was no cure, there was no hope, just get worse fast and then—

When one person is sick in a family, everyone is affected and my parents were on the front line with me. I didn't get that for a long time because I was so wrapped up in my own self-serving horror show.

At the condo, my father watched a lot of TV. If he was conscious the television was on. If it was bedtime he turned off the TV and marched straight to the bedroom with a quick pit stop at the bathroom. I used to think he was trying to get to sleep as fast as he could so that he wouldn't have to go more than five conscious minutes without the television set being on in front of him. If he wasn't watching CNN he was watching another news program. It was an exceptional occasion when a program surfaced onto his viewing schedule that was something other than the news unless it was an NFL football game. No matter what he was watching, the only time conversation would be tolerated was during a commercial break except when he liked the commercial.

He would have the television tuned to a news show and he would be reading the newspaper at the same time. There was nothing you could say to him that he didn't have an opinion on. I tried to use that as a starting point for a conversation. When CNN was running the same tape of the same story for the umpteenth time I would ask him a question about that particular issue so that he could expound on it. He liked doing that and I got to feel like we were having a conversation every now and then. News shows don't exactly lend themselves to a lot of chuckles and good humor. As a result of his obsession for being tuned into the bad news all the time, I think that added to whatever strain he put himself in.

Living with my father felt like walking on eggshells. He had two moods – okay and flaming angry. I never knew what set him off and he could change moods literally in the blink of an eye. I wouldn't have a clue what it was I had said or done to cause the latest uproar. On more than one occasion he leapt up from his La-Z-Boy, charged across the room, grabbed my wheelchair and pushed me into my bedroom door frame. I would end up in my room crying not knowing what had caused his latest outburst.

One evening, after another particularly upsetting run-in with my father, I found myself in my bedroom crying again. In the midst of all my blubbering and feeling sorry for myself, I suddenly stopped. I saw my reaction to his anger. I realized that I was in my room crying because that is what I had decided to do with his anger – be the miserable, weak, helpless, crippled child. I wanted him to feel bad for what he'd done to me so I became the victim and cried hopefully loud enough for him to hear me over the volume setting he had punched into the remote control. I wanted him to hear me and hear the upset he had caused. After realizing how useless my reaction was to his anger, my next thought was *this is stupid. Stop it.*

I turned my wheelchair around, rolled back into the living room right up to my father sitting in his easy chair and pressed the wheel-chair foot rests against his ankles so he had nowhere to go. We were knee to knee and face to face. I blocked his view of the sacred TV set. That was incredibly dangerous territory to be in but there I was, smack dab in his line of sight, interrupting his television program and trapping him in his chair.

I looked him straight in the eye and said, "I don't know what to do with you. I really truly don't."

He said nothing. I rolled back to my bedroom without another word or another tear. That was the moment I stopped being a child and started to take my life back.

Attack of Bell's Palsy

Over time, my father's humour became increasingly difficult to live with. He worked until he was seventy, a year after we moved in together at the condo. I was working for the engineering company out of the office workspace we had created in the sunroom and that's where I spent most of my time. While my father was still working, he was out of the condo during the day and it was more relaxed for my mother and I. When he retired, my parents got into the habit of going out on errands at least twice and sometimes three times a day. That's how they got their space and I got mine. When his miserable humour got to be too much for my mother, she would tell my father she was going on a window shopping expedition, something she knew he wouldn't be interested in doing. That's how she got time to herself.

It got so tense living with my parents that I decided to leave. I couldn't take living in the strained atmosphere my father created any longer. I didn't know where I was going but I had to get out of there. Maybe I could stay with a friend for a night or two until I figured out what to do.

The morning I planned to leave, I headed for the kitchen to get my breakfast when my mother told me my father hadn't been feeling well that morning. He had driven himself to the hospital. He told her he was having trouble eating breakfast so with the thought that he might be having a bit of a stroke he took himself to emergency on his way to the office.

He thought he might be having a bit of a stroke? He drove himself to emergency on his way to work? My mother didn't go with him?

I decided to wait and see what happened before I left. I still wasn't sure where I was going anyway.

My father didn't go to the office that day. When he came home from emergency he said it wasn't a stroke. After tests they told him it was Bell's palsy. He said between the time he left the condo and when he got to the hospital emergency department, the whole right side of his face had stiffened up. He said he got very prompt attention because the nurses and doctors also thought he could be having a stroke. He was shocked by everything that had happened to him that morning. He didn't turn the television on. He talked and I talked to him a lot about things I had come to understand from working with Dan and Kevin. I also gave him my own take on what was and wasn't possible in the way of treatments. Basically, I gave him a massive pep talk. The big surprise was he listened.

I had an appointment with Kevin later that afternoon and I talked to him about how awful my father's humour had become and how lousy the atmosphere in the condo was. I told him I had been planning to leave that morning. Kevin said that people who are sick will quite often exhibit changing or worsening humour. That was probably what I had witnessed with my father. Now that the illness had shown itself and been diagnosed, he suggested things would probably lighten up.

My father had been told there wasn't a lot that could be done to treat Bell's palsy. Of course, I didn't buy that and encouraged him to keep making phone calls until he found a doctor who was willing to work with him. He found a lady doctor who told him there were no guarantees but she thought they could give it a try.

The first time he saw her they had a long appointment – maybe about an hour and a half. She gave him a lot of different facial exercises he could do and suggested he buy a free-standing mirror so he could see himself doing them. Hopefully, with regular practice, he'd get the muscles that were frozen in half of his face to loosen up. She told him she was going to have some surgery done and would be unavailable for a couple of weeks but when she got back they would schedule another appointment to see what progress he'd made.

My father liked the doctor and was encouraged by her positive attitude. He got himself a good-sized free-standing mirror and did the exercises faithfully. It was going to take time but he was committed to making the effort. His humour improved and my mother and I were encouraging. Then one morning when my parents were reading the newspaper, my mother asked my father what his doctor's name was. He gave her the name and the next thing my mother said was the doctor had passed away. She handed him the section of the paper she was looking at and said the woman's picture was beside her obituary. My father took the paper, read the write up, and confirmed she was the doctor he had seen. I don't know what was more shocking – my father's Bell's palsy or that dear doctor's untimely death.

My father made phone calls to get additional confirmation that she had in fact passed away. He got a sympathy card and wrote a letter he put in it. He left the card at the doctor's office hoping it would be passed on to her family. It was and a family member called my father to thank him for the card. They were pleased to know how she had helped someone so recently. It turned out the doctor had cancer of the throat and she had passed away on the operating table. It was so sad for her and her family.

It was so sad for my father.

I had never felt sorry for him before but I did now. It was a terrible loss. He put the mirror away and within six months he had a second attack of Bell's palsy that froze the muscles in the other half of his face.

Father and Son

I think it was a combination of my father's bouts with Bell's palsy, the doctor's sudden death and having stood up to him that made me look at him differently. I started to think about the stories I'd heard since childhood about his side of the family and his experiences growing up not as separate anecdotal incidents but within a broader context of how they may have shaped his life.

I thought his father, my grandfather, was the greatest. Ganga thought I was pretty terrific, too. It was a mutual adoration society. I have never laughed so hard with anyone in my life. We brought out the most hysterically silly in each other. To this day, I remember doing a version of *'I'm a Little Teapot'* that brought the house down. He was the best audience. Sometimes, he would join in the song and sometimes he just egged me on. I didn't care which. It was too much fun having him around.

From all reports, my grandparents knew how to have a good time and were always ready for a party. They were terrific hosts. Family and friends were always welcome. One of my grandfather's sisters who they called Aunt Toon, lived nearby and when the party needed a little music they would phone her and say 'Toonie, get over here. We need a piano.' Being a good sport she always obliged. It only took her the amount of time necessary to dab a powder puff on her face once or twice and she was ready to go.

If they decided they wanted to go to a restaurant, it was always one of the better restaurants in town and my parents would get the call. I was included and set up in a high chair. My mother said there wasn't a princess who was treated better by those waiters. Those waiters also knew the princess's grandfather had a pocket full of dollar bills he generously shared when he was pleased with the service.

My father's older brother, Billy, had enlisted to fight the Nazis and was a tail gunner flying for Canada with the Alouette Squadron out of Britain. Young men who were friends of Bill's going to or coming home from the war were welcome in my grandparents' finished basement to drink and have some fun behind the blackout curtains covering the windows.

It was no secret how great I thought Ganga was and even though he had his own funny stories to tell, it must've rankled my father to hear that. The dark side of my grandfather was he was an alcoholic. My parents described him as the kind of alcoholic who could go months without a drink even if a party was going on and then one day he wouldn't come home from the office. Sometimes my grandmother wouldn't know for two or three days where he was and my mother said the dark circles under my grandmother's eyes were apparent from worrying and not sleeping. Sometimes he would go to a restaurant in Montréal called Mother Martin's where they knew him. They would call my grandmother and let her know he was there. Sometimes he would come home drunk, and stay in the basement for a lost weekend, drinking and talking to himself. My mother said you could hear him rambling from upstairs.

My mother said a lot of the men who fought in the First World War came home with drinking problems. My grandfather was under-age when he enlisted. He got as far as England before his age was discovered but when it was, he was shipped back home. The Spanish flu pandemic was in full swing by that time. It took three weeks for his ship to cross the Atlantic headed back to Canada because so many of the men onboard were sick and dying of the flu. His job on board the ship was to tend to the men who were sick and send the bodies of the dead to their final resting place at sea. He also made up the little metal boxes of personal effects so those items could be given to their families. By some miracle, my grandfather didn't get the flu.

When the Second World War ended in 1945 my father was almost seventeen. He had joined the air cadets but was too young to enlist. The years that his older brother Bill was away in England were tough for him. He missed Billy and his parents were fighting a lot. Drink was never far from the argument. There were many occasions when my father was disappointed because my grandfather didn't show up to watch him play football or see him in a hockey game. When he was sixteen he couldn't take his parents' fighting anymore and he ran away. My father always said the biggest mistake of his life was taking the train west from Montréal instead of east. He went to Toronto to an aunt and uncle who, of course, called his parents and he went back home. If he had gone east it would have been to the Maritimes and he didn't know anybody there. That would've been better. He always regretted that decision.

The stories about how tough my grandfather could be with his sons were always told by my mother and never by my father. Disciplining the boys usually involved a beating. When my grandfather was beating one son he would make the other sit there and watch. My father was apparently beaten so hard on one occasion that my grandmother didn't send him to school because of the bruises. The one thing my father did talk about was the time he flushed my grandfather's belt down the toilet. He would get a small grin on his face when he told that story. He never said a word about what kind of a beating he got after that prank but you knew my grandfather had more than one belt.

My father adored his big brother Billy and Billy was a hero to my grandparents. I never got the impression from the stories I heard that my father got as much positive attention from his parents. He probably didn't hear things like 'I love you' or 'I'm proud of you'. Hugging my father was like wrapping your arms around a tree trunk. It was alive but it was hard and didn't hug you back. I remember in high school hugging him once and he left his arms straight down at his side. It occurred to me why he never said 'I love you' or he was proud of me or 'way to go, Cath'. He didn't know how. He had no frame of reference as a parent for that kind of conversation. He never heard it so he didn't know how to say it to his own children.

After coming to that conclusion, I decided I was going to show him by example that it was okay to say things like 'I love you'. If I got the courage together to say it to him, maybe he would get used to the sound of it. Maybe he could say it back. Wouldn't it be lovely if saying 'I love you' wasn't the foreign and emotionally overwhelming brick wall it was in our household?

The Boulder-sized
Bread Crumb

On more than one occasion Kevin told me when I was ready to accept the responsibility things would change with the MS. Well, hell. I'm responsible. I pay my taxes, I go to the dentist regularly, and I return phone calls.

I'm knocking myself out here.

How much more responsible could I be?

(*Loud, rude noise*). Thank you for playing. Try again.

One day Kevin loaned me a three-tape video set he had called *The Biology of Belief.* The tapes showed this fellow, Dr. Bruce Lipton, lecturing to students. At least I assumed they were students of some sort. I guessed they could have been chiropractic students because the tape came from Kevin but I don't really know. The lecture was about how cells are affected by our thoughts and how the mechanics work between the cell in the body and the brain and thought.

Fascinating.

What I found particularly enjoyable about this Dr. Lipton was his enthusiasm. He was so full of energy. He had a big smile on his face and he was absolutely thrilled to share his ideas and under-standings. He talked like he had just made the discoveries and couldn't contain his excitement; he was bursting with the news. It was infectious.

In the middle of watching the second tape for the second time, that word 'responsibility' kept going through my mind.

Weird…

The man is talking cells and how thoughts affect them and I'm sitting here with the word 'responsibility' going through my head.

I watched all three videotapes again and slowly but surely under-standing started to seep into my bones. As the fog was lifting I began to see how I saw my world. It was emotions and mostly hidden, angry ones. It was intellectual where I made contact with the outside world but physical? I saw my body as the necessary vehicle that got my head and wounded heart from point A to point B. But apparently there was a much more intimate and powerful connection between the three parts than just keeping the body tuned up with a health club membership.

Whatever I was thinking or feeling could physically affect my cells and their subsequent relationship to my body. It wasn't just my mind or my emotions operating separately from each other and from me physically. I began to see that I had spent a great chunk of my life operating separately from myself physically. To me, what I had iden-tified as the Inside Me, repetitive mind-movies and emotions, I saw as operating completely separately from me physically. Emotions and thoughts had absolutely nothing to do with my body. The Inside Me had nothing to do with the Outside Me. I hadn't seen a relation-ship between those aspects until now. And when I finally saw it, it was so blatantly obvious.

Rise and shine, Cathy. Connect the dots.

Whenever Dan was about to say something to me that he knew I would have to brace myself for he would start by saying, "Are you sitting down?" Funny guy. But it's a good thing I was sitting down when thoughts-cells-responsibility-martyr-heroine-body-affect-MS hit.

For years, I was flaming angry and my self-esteem was the stuff of bottom-feeders. The Martyr Heroine ruled a huge chunk of my waking thoughts. If all those miserable movie scenarios I replayed continually in my mind affected my cells and how they functioned then I could easily have been in a weakened state susceptible to some kind of physical breakdown. After all, how much bashing with negative thinking could a cell take? I not only had a phenomenal amount of ground to make up to correct the damage my Martyr Heroine thinking had done to my mindset but these tapes may have also given me a large part of the answer as to why I had MS. And if indeed that was the case that I had beaten myself up for so long I had made myself available to illness, then why MS? Why not some other illness? If I could beat a cell to a buttery pulp with constant negative thinking, then could I end the illness and return to health with relentless positive practice? Why not? Anything is possible, right?

If I thought negatively would I automatically create disease? What I understood from the tapes was continual negative thinking could be a contributing factor that could have left me physically weakened with an immune system that had been compromised so many times I was wide open to hosting a disease. I could have kicked away any defenses I had around my weakest link so that try as it might, my body couldn't take one more miserable thought.

I could keep all the appointments in the world, answer every phone call and show up on time with my taxes but if I didn't show up for *me*, then I was missing the biggest piece of what it meant to be responsible. I could always reschedule an appointment, return a phone call later, or pay interest on my taxes for late filing but the one thing I couldn't put off was backing me up.

Standing up for me equals true responsibility.

Kevin had been trying to teach me that it was all right to say what I wanted or needed, that the world didn't end when I spoke up for myself. I didn't dare ask for what I really wanted because from the time I was a youngster I had always felt that my requests were unwelcome impositions. I got that message from my father. Growing up I started to censor myself so I wouldn't be disappointed. I should have been more rebellious as a teenager.

Segment 8 – You are an Entity

You are an entity

passing through a life

in which the entire life drama

is a feeding for

your awakening.

Ram Dass
Grist for the Mil

The "F" Word

I have help for which I am very grateful because I need assistance with everything from getting in and out of bed to getting my shoes on, but there are times when communicating directions for what I need help with goes beyond English and my catalogue of synonyms and goes beyond my strength to repeat instructions one more time, in spite of the addition of hand signals. When I feel like I'm duct-taped to teeth-gnashing frustration and annoyed beyond description at my failure to get the help I need to complete an otherwise simple task, that's when I do my salute to Edvard Munch and perform my version of *The Scream*. I take a deep breath, close my eyes tightly, open my mouth wide, strain all the muscles in my face and pretend to scream for all I'm worth. I know it's childish but when I exhale and relax I feel so much better. Then I try to get my point across again, hopefully in a different and more successful way.

Frustration is first cousin to that other "F" word. Sometimes I think they are synonymous. There are two kinds of frustration. There is the frustration of trying to be understood by someone else – a Well Person. And then there is the frustration of me working with myself.

Examples of how I frustrate myself would include not being able to do up buttons on a blouse, hold a pen well enough to write, and because of a minor tremor I have in my right hand, holding cutlery in my left. That allows me to regularly slide food off my fork on to the floor.

When I was a Well Person it was easy to toss off a remark and have it understood or at least I thought it was understood by another Well Person and I could do the same for them. It was so fast. But communicating from a wheelchair can be very slow and tedious because of the need to be precise when speaking with someone who is not only able-bodied but whose mind is a firecracker of instant messaging. Communicating with the able world oftentimes pushes me into a state of impatience.

Hey, people. I used to speak Well Person just like you.

I had no idea how challenging communication would become as my MS graduated from stumbling to a wheelchair. The biggest part of the communication snafus I experienced seemed to be how Well People only heard what I was saying in fragments and taking those fragments they jumped to conclusions. I began to think that the speed at which a Well Person can process even partial fragments of information was amazing. All those spaces between words that are actually spoken and the subtext of words not spoken but whose meanings are implied can produce conclusions that aren't anywhere near what is intended. I could see a Well Person's brain snapping, hissing and sparking as they took in their surroundings, circum-stances and my fragmented information about the task at hand.

For example:

WP: Where do you keep your vegetable peeler?

Me: It's in the dr—

Well Person opens fridge.

Me: It's in the dr—

Well Person opens cupboard.

 Me: No, it's—

Well Person moves towards sink. I cry out.

Me: Stop. Turn around. It's in the dr—

Well Person opens drawer in counter and produces vegetable peeler.

WP: Got it.

When I was first living with my parents in the condo, I would be trying to figure out how to do something but my parents expected me to give them the answer for how to do it before I had figured it out. At first I thought it was just my parents and they were impatient, but over time I realized their reaction was the same for most Well People. They would give me three seconds and one try to get something done for the first time, and if I didn't accomplish what I was aiming for, then they jumped in and did it for me. If I stopped them because I wanted to try a second time, Well People generally got ticked off because I wasn't letting them help me. They would be ticked off at me. I would be ticked off at them and the frustration level amped up another notch.

And then there are the occasions where the person who is helping me will understand what it is I've asked them to do but they will make a different and unilateral decision. For example, a Well Person will come in the door holding a piece of paper they took from my mailbox and ask, "Where do you want this?" I'll say, "You can leave it right there on the table." The Well Person will turn around, walk in the opposite direction and leave it on the kitchen counter saying there's more room for it there than on the table.

Directions can be tricky. Up and down, stop and go are generally understood but what I may have to do is repeat the instruction two or three times to confirm I know what I'm talking about. Left and right are much more difficult concepts. I've learned to give a landmark, thereby creating the direction in which I want some action to go. For example, if I'd like my foot moved to the left, I'll suggest that this foot needs to go over to the lamp beside the bed.

When the MS first started to make itself known, it was scary because one hour would be different from the next. I didn't know what was coming and I couldn't plan for it. One minute I would feel like an overcooked noodle and the next minute I'd be fine. As the world I was used to living in became harder to manage, my frustration grew. I wondered if it was ever going to end and feared it never would.

If I was having a bad day, I got to the point where I could say, 'Okay, it's a bad day' and give myself permission to feel lousy and hopeless. From experience, I learned the next day always brought something new. Pretty soon even the bad days started to lighten up. The frustration would still flare from time to time but I started to forgive myself for having those crummy moments, too. I learned to relax sooner and became more confident in my belief that something else was on its way, probably something better. I just had to pay attention and watch for it.

The Cane

Years after I had walked away from the traditional Western medical establishment, my father found a neurologist I liked. She didn't check her watch and then cast a sorrowful look in my direction. She referred to dealing with MS as managing. "How shall we manage what we have?" she asked. That was a more positive attitude than I had met with before. So I came out of the woodwork, stopped hiding and excusing my symptoms and went through the testing that would forever brand me as having a chronic illness. By doing that, I officially signed up with a neurologist and that was the key to opening a treasure trove of government programs, assistance and access to equipment. I had no idea that was how the system worked. However, for the job of getting the Sunday newspaper off the top of my fridge, there was a simple piece of equipment I had already purchased all by myself – a cane.

Well People, I discovered, like to put things up high. One of their favourite places to put things is the top of the fridge. When I moved to the co-op, the top of my fridge became a popular site for coffee cups, keys, pop bottles and mail. This was fascinating to me because even when I was healthy and had my own place to live, I never put anything on top of my fridge. In thirty years of having my own fridge, it never occurred to me but now I was living in a place where aide workers were available to help those of us with disabilities. If I was looking for something and I thought it might've been handled last by an aide, a Well Person, I went to the kitchen and looked up. Nine times out of ten I found what I was looking for on top of the fridge.

This particular Sunday morning I was looking for my newspaper. I rolled my wheelchair all over the apartment and looked. I looked outside in the hallway. I was about to go downstairs to see if the newspapers had been left inside the lobby when I remembered to go to the kitchen and look up. There was a small corner of the newspaper hanging over the top of the fridge.

Perfect. Now what?

How do I get it down from there, I wondered. That's when I remembered the cane. I hadn't used it since I got the wheelchair but I hadn't gotten rid of it either. I got it out of the front hall closet. I used the rubber end of the cane to prod the underside of the newspaper corner that was hanging over the edge of the fridge. One careful, gentle nudge at a time I moved the newspaper until finally it fell onto my lap, sections intact and in order. Now that's what I call managing a situation.

Another instance of problem solving with my cane involved a new baby potato. I love new baby potatoes. When they became available in summer I usually purchase a small bag of them. On this particular occasion I decided to boil four of them for dinner that night. One of the new baby potatoes fell on the floor and rolled to the wall underneath the kitchen counter. At first I tried to roll it back to me using a dishtowel but rather than the material catching it, the towel rolled the little potato farther away. Then I thought of the cane.

Holding the rubber end, I used the cane handle to corral the potato and bring it towards me. When it was close enough I reached to pick it up but the tremor in my hand inadvertently pushed the potato away again. Time after time I corralled the new baby potato with the cane handle but when I reached for it my hand spasm sent the lively little potato rolling away.

My personal care attendant for that meal service arrived to help me put dinner together. She saw what I was trying to do and immediately stepped forward to pick up the potato. After all of my effort there was no way some Well Person was going to steal my moment of success. I told the aide I would get it. I was determined. I knew I could do it. I wanted that accomplishment. I deserved it. She reached towards the potato a second time. I told her to stop, I could do it. She backed off and watched. I missed again but I was getting closer. I tried one more time and at the same moment she stepped forward to get the potato. I swung the cane along the floor and stopped just short of hitting her feet. "Oh," she gasped and jumped back. I told her picking up the potato meant nothing to her but it meant a lot to me. I told her I had been working at it diligently. I knew I could do it and the accomplishment of picking it up belonged to me. She looked at me like I was speaking a foreign language but she stayed back.

Well People can take a step, reach forward and pick something up with effort so minimal a split second later they don't remember what they just did. It's thoughtless action. But to me picking up that new baby potato with a wonky hand while bending over from a wheelchair was a huge accomplishment. I was not about to let her snatch that moment away from me. And she didn't.

I picked up the potato, put it in the pot of boiling water, scooped it out with a strainer when it was cooked, put it on my plate with a little butter and black pepper and I ate the sucker.

Independence Day

An occupational therapist came to the condo ono day with a small three-wheel scooter for me to try. It was intended to be used indoors getting around the condo. If the condo had been Buckingham Palace with long, wide hallways this little scooter would have been handy but our place wasn't that big, never mind trying to get around the furniture we had packed into it. What I really wanted to do was get it outside and take it for a spin down the street. The therapist wasn't keen on that idea. He felt a small three-wheel scooter would not be that great on uneven pavement. Sidewalk curb cuts could definitely tip it over but after some prodding he relented.

We took the elevator to the underground garage, hit the button to open the garage doors and out I drove, up the ramp to the sidewalk. I was all ready to go on my adventure but the therapist figured I had gone about as far as I should go on that piece of equipment. So I just sat on the scooter on the sidewalk and imagined the freedom it could bring me.

Darn. I was that close to freedom.

Later that week at a barbecue, I told my former boss about the scooter and what a thrill it was to ride it as far as the sidewalk from the garage. He was really interested and said that he and his partner had been trying to figure out something they could do for me and a scooter sounded like a great idea. A few days later I was in his car and we were heading for a medical supply store that also sold scooters.

There were various models of scooters in a row inside the store. The salesman pulled one from the line-up so it was facing me as I sat in my wheelchair. I said, "Oh my gosh, it's got a headlight." Very seriously the salesman turned the headlight on and said "And it's got signal lights." He flipped a couple of switches and the headlight stayed on with the yellow bulb on the right side flashing. Then the yellow bulb on the left side started to go. He said "It's got hazard lights, too" and pressed another button. The scooter lit up with lights flashing at the front and the rear. I burst out laughing.

I was imagining scooting down the sidewalk, running into a problem, pulling over to the inside and flipping on the hazard lights. Better caution all oncoming pedestrians that my vehicle is experiencing mechanical difficulties.

What a hoot.

I couldn't believe it. The salesman wanted to demonstrate some other scooter models but I wanted that one. It lit up like the fireworks on Canada Day and it was cherry red to boot. You couldn't beat that combination.

I got on the scooter and we went outside. I rode around the parking lot with my boss sort of jogging alongside. I wasn't actually going as fast as it felt I was. We even crossed the street. It was fantastic. When we were finished with our test drive, my boss asked the salesman for a bigger basket at the front of the scooter than the little dinky toy one it came with. The salesman obliged and my boss double checked that red was the color I wanted. The salesman said he would bring it out to the condo that afternoon.

Driving back to my place looking out the car window, I was so overwhelmed by the possibilities and freedom the scooter represented that I was dizzy. Every place I saw going by I could get to now. Where I had felt so confined by the condo and trapped in the wheelchair, suddenly everything opened up and I could get anywhere I wanted to go. My brains went on tilt and I was dizzy looking out the car window.

The scooter gave me mobility. It gave me the opportunity to re-educate my sight. When I was on the scooter everything I saw was either new or I saw it from a completely different perspective than I had seen it before. It occurred to me that I had adjusted to the MS in a thousand little incremental ways, progressively moving in one downward direction. When I got the scooter, those tiny little downward increments began to move in the opposite direction. One direction isn't better than the other. The downward movement provided massive amounts of learning. But the upward progressive perspective that was now being created by riding the scooter came with joy. Instead of frustration there was discovery. Instead of worry there was problem solving. Where there was coping there were now possibilities.

The result of all this movement over bridges, along city streets, in and out of the river valley, on buses and light rail transit coaches, in and out of stores, meeting friends for restaurant lunches made me feel like something had shaken loose – it was probably my concept of myself as a person with a disability. Profound thanks go to my two former bosses. You know not what you created.

Butts and Belt Buckles

Imagine being in a wheelchair in the middle of a crowd of sixteen thousand people all trying to exit a concert venue at the same time. I see a wall of backs and butts. Just how does your butt look in your jeans? I can tell you. The view from my scooter riding along the sidewalk is about the same except I can also see oncoming belt buckles. I look for spaces between jean labels so I can scoot past Well People who are in my path. Let me reassure you, the ones who look good in their jeans are the exceptions. Most everybody – male and female – could use a little work.

Well People's point of view of me is the space about a foot above my head. I see their lower forty and they see my upper space. They only see the space above my head because I'm below their line of sight. If a Well Person is six feet tall and they're standing up looking straight ahead, their point of view is six feet tall. Sitting in my wheelchair or on my scooter I'm probably five feet plus an inch or two. The discrepancy between me and a six-foot tall Well Person is the space above my head. Ergo, I am a space. I don't exist to a six foot tall Well Person unless they are approaching me from a distance, in which case I have entered their visual range.

I saw a program about wildlife and how predators determine what is prey. If something alive and moving is below a predator's line of sight, that moving object could be dinner. You know those orange triangle flags atop skinny sticks that are attached to wheelchairs and scooters? Those flags are there to startle a Well Person by unexpectedly flapping orange smack dab in their line of sight so they will think, "Hey. What the – oh yeah, a scooter."

Well People are surprised when they happen to look down and suddenly realize I have materialized in front of them. Sometimes they walk right into me especially if they have just bolted out of a door walking in one direction but looking in another. It's fascinating. I think *they* think it makes them look busy, like they're doing two things at once – walking in one direction but looking in another. I was probably one of those Well People BMS (before MS).

And then there are the people who text. When I see one of those people coming at me, head down, focused on their palm-sized keyboard, I simply stop and watch them continue to march straight at me. Just as they are about to kick the scooter, they look up. They usually gasp, say a quick 'sorry', step to the side and keep going, head down, still texting. They make me chuckle.

When I was riding horses, I learned that if I looked at where I wanted to go I would better direct the horse because I would automatically shift my body weight and use my hands on the reins in a way that let the horse know where I was headed. So it helped to think of my scooter as a horse. The incidents of Well People careening into me on my scooter because they bolted out of a doorway without paying attention to what direction their body was going, even though their eyes were looking the other way, never mind seeing me in their path, don't happen that often. I see what they're doing before they hit me. Moving on a crowded sidewalk I'm patient and wait for my opportunities. I pick my moments to scoot between jean labels and make progress on my own journey. I also try to avoid crowds.

Wheelchair 101

Well People push wheelchairs like they are strollers and just like a baby in a stroller, I have no control over where I'm going and everything of interest happens behind me. When I walked, I could go to the entrance of a store, take one look around and see if there was a rack of clothes or something interesting on a countertop that caught my interest enough to actually go into the store and shop. If nothing caught my eye, I went on to the next store. Once I was in the wheelchair, I couldn't see around clothes racks never mind see what was on the top of a counter even if I was parked right beside it. When I'm in my wheelchair in a store, I'm dependent on the person who is pushing the chair to get me where I think I want to go so I can see what it is I have in mind to look at.

Clothes racks are the stuff of mazes for me. Stores are labyrinths and clothes racks are the corn stalks I can't see above or around. If I suddenly come into an aisle that is wide enough and allows me to see ahead, I feel like the explorer who has whacked her way through dense jungle to a clearing. I can see where it is I want to go.

"Over there. The slacks are over there."

I point and call to my companion pushing the wheelchair. My companion, who has also had the same moment of being in a merchandising gap, will answer my cry of discovery with, "Jackets. I need a new spring jacket." And while I'm looking one way pointing at the slacks, the wheelchair swings around and once again I am charging through the clothes rack maze away from my wardrobe needs. Maybe I will get lucky as we're leaving the store and accidentally bump into the rack of slacks that caught my eye for that one brief shining moment.

Sometimes, when a Well Person is pushing the wheelchair down an aisle lined with shelving, they will see something on display that catches their eye. They will stop the wheelchair, pick up the item and say, "Look at this. Isn't it great?" They are behind me. I am in front of them and pointed in the direction we are traveling, looking down the aisle ahead of us. They have picked something off a shelf which is behind me. I have already been pushed past it. They are admiring an item I have already gone by. The first few times this happened when I wanted to know what they were talking about, I wrenched myself around in the chair so I could look backwards and see. I stopped doing that because Linda Blair impersonations were hard to do. Instead, I would remain looking straight ahead and say something like, "Oh, gee, that's great." The Well Person pushing the chair would realize I hadn't turned around to look and, in fact, they were behind me. Then they would bring the item of interest around to my front so I could take a look at it. That was so much easier on me.

The baby-in-a-stroller wheelchair pushing phenomenon happens generally with women who have raised children. For instance, I will be pushed into a waiting room at a medical office and stopped beside a seat they sit in but my wheelchair won't be turned around. I'm parked facing the wall. They can look at me or the rest of the waiting room. I can look at them or the wall. The rest of the waiting room, reception desk, clock, and magazines are all behind me.

When the receptionist calls my name and I answer that I'm here, I have my back to them and I'm talking to the wall.

Another aspect of the baby-in-a-stroller phenomenon happens when I'm meeting friends outside a building. Happy to see them as I'm being pushed closer to the group I wave and call out, "Hi."

When we get to where the group is standing, suddenly my wheelchair is swung around so the Well Person who pushed me there is standing with the group but I'm looking at the parking lot. I watch a few cars go by and when I'm sure the Well Person who pushed me there has let go of the chair, I take hold of the wheels and turn the chair around so I can participate in the conversation.

No wonder babies in strollers get cranky.

Little Boys and Old Men

One of the best things about being on a scooter is little boys. I mean truly little boys – under three years of age. I have come to the conclusion that their reaction to seeing the scooter is genetic. Little boys don't see the space a foot above my head. They're too short. In fact, they rarely see me at all. What they see is the scooter and they are filled with wonder and awe, with rabid respect washing over their gleaming eyes.

I met my mother for lunch one day in a restaurant. She had gotten there ahead of me and was already seated at a table beside a young professional couple who were having lunch with their little boy seated in a chair with a booster seat. I'd say he was maybe a year and a half. He was sitting up very well in his chair and was meticulously eating Cheerios one at a time from the line of tasty toasted O's that had been put on the table in front of him. I eased the scooter into position beside the table where my mother sat. The little boy turned holding a Cheerio in midair halfway to his open mouth. He froze in that position at the sight of the scooter next to him. I could see his mind working – *"It's got wheels, it's got lights, it's cherry apple red and it moves. I want one."*

I was at a wedding parked in the space between the pew and the wall of the church. In the middle of the ceremony I looked down to see a little boy standing beside the scooter, his right hand on the arm of the chair, his left hand on the scooter's handlebar. He looked up at me with an expression that asked if it was okay for him to touch. I leaned down to him and whispered, "Do you like bikes?" He squatted and very gently touched the tread on the rear tire with one pudgy index finger. He looked up again and this time the expression in his eyes said he couldn't believe it. His father came along crouching low behind the scooter, took the little boy's hand and quietly led his son back to their seats.

In a bookstore, a little boy with a soother in his mouth made a noise to catch his mother's attention when he saw me and pointed at the scooter. He walked over and put his hand on the round yellow turning light. I flipped the switch and the beeping noise sounded at the same time as the yellow light flashed. He startled and pulled his hand away. I flipped the switch again so the yellow light on the other side of the scooter started to flash. He looked up at his mother to make sure she was watching and when he turned back to look at the scooter he was grinning – the soother clenched tight between his teeth.

Male retirees will see me coming and stop in their tracks to watch. When I am just about to pass them they will say something and their questions will generally go in the same order:

How fast does that go?

How much does it cost?

How far can you go?

You plug it in?

They want one.

When I'm on my scooter headed eastbound on the sidewalk and I'm about to pass a male retiree on a scooter headed westbound, the male retiree will always give a little nod acknowledging a comrade as he passes. It's kind of like being part of the brotherhood of scooters. We recognize each other.

Male retirees are very open to the possibility of using a scooter even if they can still walk. Female retirees use walkers. They struggle with groceries and they struggle with errands. Male retirees can't be bothered putting up with a walker when they could get on a scooter and cover a lot more ground faster.

A female retiree stopped me one day outside Safeway. She had just finished her shopping and was sitting on the seat of her walker. She was loaded down with grocery bags and she was obviously tired. The seniors' residence she lived in was across the street but for her at the end of her shopping tour that was still a long way to go. She had to get to the corner, wait for a green light to cross the intersection and walk another half a block to the door of her apartment building.

She looked at me on the scooter and said her doctor was encouraging her to buy one of those things but she just didn't know. I told her all about it and said if she could afford to buy one, a scooter was well worth the investment. I told her about the store where I got mine and the fact that they had sales every now and then. She should watch for one. She still wasn't convinced when I left but there she was – tired and sitting on her walker. She's the only female retiree who has ever stopped me to talk about the scooter.

The scooter is definitely a boy thing. It doesn't matter how old they are, their reaction is genetic – it's got wheels, it flashes, it moves, and you ride it. The older boys think *"I'm not getting gouged at the pumps. I plug it in and go."* And it's cherry apple red. It doesn't get much better than that.

Girls don't know what they're missing.

Happy Guts

A friend dropped by the condo with a booklet he got from an acupuncturist we both knew. She had given it to him to pass along to me. The booklet was written by a naturopath in California detailing her program for treating multiple sclerosis by following the Candida diet. Apparently, the naturopath had healed her own MS with this diet. I hadn't tried diet as a way to ease the symptoms of MS. I had only used supplements and different modalities like acupuncture or massage. Revamping my diet was a new idea and I figured I might as will give it a try.

The naturopath divided foods into what worked and what didn't in terms of Candida and alleviating MS symptoms. Her list of foods that didn't work, I either didn't like or only ate occasionally. The foods she listed that were of benefit I generally liked. The only thing I knew I was going to have a problem with was she said to eliminate bread, flour, and pasta. Like the song says, these were a few of my favourite things.

Oh well, maybe I could work around that.

I followed her suggestions for a while and I started to feel better but even though some things improved I didn't realize I was still making mistakes in terms of food choices.

I told another friend who had diagnosed herself with Candida some years before that I was following the Candida diet. By trial and error and with the good things she grew in her fabulous garden she cured herself of the condition. It took a while but she did it. She had all sorts of helpful suggestions to make including finding a naturopath who could give me homeopathic drops that would further clear the toxins out of my body. I found a naturopath, got the drops and started to clean up the evil toxins I apparently had.

My body's reaction to the drops was to break out in circular, brownish, dime-sized spots on my arms and legs. It took a couple of days for the spots to form. They would be there for a few days and then they would fade away. My friend said that was a sign that the toxins were leaving my system. As my diet improved I got fewer spots but as soon as I ate something I shouldn't according to the diet, the spots were back.

Another friend I had known since grade one was an avid proponent of eating wheat and gluten-free based on her personal experience of raising three wheat-sensitive children. She had educated herself reading everything she could from books on allergies to product labels. She had been on at me for years about avoiding wheat and gluten. When I told her about the funny reaction I was having to the homeopathic drops, her immediate response was, "It's the gluten. It's not just wheat. The basmati rice you're devouring? It has gluten. The spelt bread you're enjoying so much – it has gluten. You have to stop eating gluten."

Yeah, yeah, yeah. I heard that before.

I had always ignored her theories because I couldn't imagine living life without bread or pasta. What kind of a life was that?

She offered name brands and manufacturers for specific products I could look for in the health food store. So I did and I came up with substitutes for foods that I liked that were pretty good. I would phone her and ask what she was cooking for dinner that night so I could get some ideas for meals that would be diet approved. I was trying to figure out how to change what was in my cupboards and fridge so I could reach for things without it being such a job to think about three times a day. Eventually, I got to the point where I was pretty much eating wheat-free and gluten-free.

After eating like that for about six months, I had lunch one day with a fellow I used to work with. We went to a restaurant that made thin crust pizzas that were delicious. He ordered one and I thought what the heck – it's a thin crust and it's been six months. So I ordered one, too. Lunch went down beautifully and gosh, it was good. Maybe I really didn't have sensitivity to gluten after all. Maybe I had cured myself of the Candida. I felt exonerated and ended the day on that happy note.

Victory

When I woke up the next morning I felt miserable. I felt miserable just like when the MS was new and came on like gangbusters. I was exhausted. I had the strength of an over-cooked noodle and my brains were wrapped in cotton balls. When the personal care attendant arrived to help me get out of bed she asked, "What's the matter with you?" Smiling, I happily told her "I ate a pizza. I thought the thin crust would make a difference but it didn't. Wheat is wheat and I shouldn't have eaten it. I feel absolutely-MS-lousy." Still lying in bed I raised my arms and looked at them. "And I've got spots. Isn't that great?"

I did some reading and found out the immune system is located in our guts. If our guts are clogged with wheat and sticky gluten that our bodies aren't prepared to handle, then the immune system can't operate properly. They call MS an autoimmune disease. Maybe this was a big chunk of what was going on with me. I experimented with the pizza to find out if it would affect me and boy, did it ever. I felt like I was on the cutting edge of science. I had proven to myself that eating something incorrectly had a terrific effect on my state of wellness or lack thereof. It was a crude trial-and-error experiment but now I had something solid to work with.

Four months later I repeated the delicious pizza experiment. I enjoyed myself immensely and the next day felt totally wrecked with the spots back on my arms. I had my answer. It may not be the whole answer but I was on the right track for sure.

I made an appointment with my GP and got a blood test to see if I had celiac. The answer was no, I didn't have celiac but what I probably did have was a sensitivity to gluten that I needed to pay attention to. Maybe I had an allergy to wheat. Maybe it was just a lifetime of eating lots of bread and pasta and my body had had enough. Maybe gluten sensitivity didn't cause MS but it sure as heck didn't help. It was really easy after that to avoid wheat and learn what else gluten was in. When I heard comments from friends and family saying, "Don't you miss it?" The answer was *no*. I don't miss feeling lousy and impersonating a slug. I don't miss cotton ball brains. I miss my legs and if skipping a pizza helps get them back in working order, so be it.

Three cheers for brown rice penne.

Fifty

I loved turning fifty. It was as if a switch had been flipped in my brain and all of the things I had worried about, anguished over losing, and been fearful of revealing my life to be a colossal failure, simply melted away. None of the things I had desperately hung onto and thought were inextricable to my personal happiness seemed to hardly matter now. It wasn't like I didn't care anymore about anything. I did care but the importance and value I attributed to hanging on to every last little bit of my life before MS shifted. The anxiety diminished. There was a great chunk of my former life I didn't have to get all hot and bothered about anymore. Were those parts of my old world important? They were yesterday but today I was fifty and I was looking at wonderful new ideas to care about. My brains changed channels and the things that I had tried to hang onto so hard for so long were still there but the intensity of hanging onto everything the way it used to be faded.

Thank God. What a relief.

Turning fifty was also a surprise. It wasn't like I thought I'd never make it to that birthday but my forties weren't a lot of laughs. From having a hysterectomy at forty-one to getting a diagnosis of primary progressive MS at forty-two to reverting to the child again living with my parents at forty-four, there were days I was so overwhelmed with fear and loss that seeing light at the end of the tunnel was out of the question. Then one morning I woke up and I was fifty.

When we're teenagers we get information by osmosis and understand things instantly that are important to our world – music, fads and fashion. It's as if just by breathing we know everything we need to know. Then we get into our twenties and we're still pretty much plugged in and we have the energy to do anything we want to do. We can do it all. We are legal. We are bulletproof. Somewhere along the line in our twenties we begin to carve out who we think we are and how we think we want our lives to be. In our thirties we think we're done. We've made all the big decisions and now it's just a matter of playing it out.

If it hasn't happened before then, the first reality bites occur – the death of a parent, a divorce, illness, losing a job. That's when we begin to think perhaps our lives aren't working out exactly the way we thought they would. We're distracted and off course from where we think we should be and we struggle to get back on track. We find ourselves wondering – how did *that* happen?

In my forties, when I was looking for someone or something to blame for my predicament, I began to wish someone had said to me, "Follow your heart" when I was a child. I thought if someone had said that to me as a little girl it could have made a world of difference to how my life developed. If someone had said, "Follow your heart", I probably could have avoided MS. Nobody told me and look at the mess I was in. But then, if someone had told me, would I have heard it? And if I had heard it would I have listened? If I had listened would I have done it?

I do wish when I was young someone had said to me, "Listen to your heart. Your heart is talking to you. You know what you feel comfortable with and what you don't. That's your heart talking to you. Listen to it. When you hear it, follow it and you will never go wrong. If you follow your heart it's impossible to get lost and confused." Why didn't somebody tell me it was not only okay to listen to my heart but it was absolutely essential to act on what it said. I wish someone had told me about the importance of personal choices and how they create a life. I could have created such a different one. But no, no one said that to me, so I didn't know. I was a tragedy waiting to happen and by golly... Well, I decided, if no one gave me that advice as a child then I would say it to me *now* as a grown-up and yes, I could follow my heart sitting in a wheelchair. I was still here, so it wasn't too late.

And I could spread the message. I started writing "Follow your heart" in birthday cards to my friends' kids. If I had gotten married and had a family, my kids would be the same ages as theirs. They would've been getting learner's permits for driving, going to the prom, graduating high school, moving on to further education or stepping out into the world. If I didn't have my own children then I could say 'follow your heart' to these kids who I had known since before they were twinkles in their parents' eyes.

It felt good to pass it on. It didn't matter that nobody said it to me as a kid. It was up to me to say it to myself now. Listen to my heart, hear it, follow it, be true to it, and be true to me. That's integrity. That's my job in this life – listen to my heart, pay attention and follow where it leads. Simple. Not always easy but simple.

Focus and discipline would create structure, Dan advised. A building can sustain damage. Wind can lift shingles. Fences lean. Paint peels. Pipes freeze. Shifting ground can crack concrete sidewalks and inattention and neglect can magnify wear and tear. I thought about the damage my body had sustained over the years, damage that I inflicted on myself: smoking, drinking more than I should have, indiscriminate and meaningless sex, unreasonable levels of work-related and self-inflicted stress, rampant self pity, unchecked martyrdom and incredible anger. My physical body took hit after hit over many years. That much accumulated damage, I believe, helped to create my MS. A virus, bacteria or other environmental factor may also have contributed but that's for the research scientists to work out.

I've thrown away a lot of soggy tissues in my time but I'm learning. When things don't go the way I think they should, I'm learning that usually means it's better if it happens another way. If I insist it has to be the way I imagined it should be, I'm learning that attitude creates unwanted aggravation. So I try to pay attention and trust that sometimes things are happening much better than I could have imagined. In his song, *Lovers in a Dangerous Time*, the wonderful Bruce Cockburn wrote the lyric "kick at the darkness till it bleeds daylight". That line describes me in my forties. I was flailing in the dark hoping to get lucky and hit a light switch. At fifty, I relaxed and heard my heart. I was sitting in a wheelchair but the Universe heard it, too, and instead of a light switch it created the horizon with a sunrise.

Segment 9 – God does not play Dice

At any rate, I am convinced that He (God) does not play dice.

Albert Einstein

Resistance

I have the 1988 edition of Louise Hay's *Heal Your Body*. It is commonly referred to as the 'Blue Book' and I have kept it on my night table since I purchased it. All these years later the book continues to be a reference for me because no matter what condition or ailment I'm looking up, Louise's explanation always gives me something to think about. In her dedication for this edition she writes, "I have long believed the following: 'Everything I need to know is revealed to me.' 'Everything I need comes to me...' There is no new knowledge. All is ancient and infinite." In the foreword she continues, "This little book does not heal anyone. It does awaken within you the ability to contribute to your own healing process."

When I was diagnosed with MS in 1995 one of the first things I did was look up the little Blue Book for Louise's probable cause for MS. For the first time since I owned the book, her explanation left me completely clueless. I didn't understand how her probable cause explanation had anything to do with me. Her probable cause said I was hard-headed, hard-hearted, had an iron will, was inflexible, and fearful.

Really?

I could look up ailments and conditions that other people had and completely understand what she was talking about but when it came to me and MS she might as well have been talking to a wall. I was in the middle of the deepest, darkest forest. A thundering herd of trees attacking me with their flailing branches would still have been a mystery to me.

Trees? What trees?

I remember vehemently making a case against Louise's probable cause for MS in a session with Dan. That was when my intellect was razor-sharp, nimble and not connected to anything but the sound of my own voice.

One day during my morning meditation, the word *resistance* careened across my mind with stunning clarity, and in the same moment I could actually feel how strong the force of my resistance could be. No sooner had the impact of slamming into my own brick wall hit my bones than my second understanding of the day revealed itself.

I don't have the courage to receive my blessings.

Receiving my blessings is not the same as *accepting* them. I can accept my blessings just fine. Yup, there they are. All lined up over there in a neat row. Those are the blessings. Yes sir, that's them.

But I didn't *receive* them. I didn't pick them up in both hands and hold them to my nose so I could breathe deep and take in their luscious fragrance. I didn't breathe in with joy and I didn't exhale with gratitude, excited because I truly knew they were mine.

So – what does a person do who is hard-headed, hard-hearted, has an iron will, is inflexible, and fearful I asked myself that morning?

'Change' was the answer that came back.

There were times when I wanted to change things in my life but I never seemed to know what I wanted to change things to. If I let go of something what would I get to replace it? I always thought it was up to me to figure out what to do next and the truth was I didn't *know* what to do next. So I stayed stuck where I was and I resented it. And the resentment grew. I always thought it was resentment towards some-thing or some-body but the truth of it was I resented me. I resented my inability to act but rather than understand and accept who I was most angry at, I stayed stuck wallowing in my miserable anger and looked for some-thing or some-body else to blame.

If I could receive my blessings, what would those blessings bring to my life?

Change.

Change isn't safe. Wallowing in my own self-imposed drama was much safer because it was familiar and I was addicted to feeling bad. Staying stuck felt safe and it fed my addiction.

Change is frightening. It's much easier to be mentally hard, hard-hearted, have a will of iron and be inflexible. With those qualities I could easily fight change but when the need for change became greater than what I could stop, I broke. And I still didn't get how this could be happening to me.

My legs didn't work. I lost my health. I lost my job. I lost my income. When I had to move in with my parents because I needed their help with daily living, I lost my home and my independence. It turned out loss was the only change I was willing to make. Now that's the definition of resistance.

And then one day I was in a session with Kevin. We hadn't really started yet but I think I had brought something to the office to show him and I remember after I gave it to him he said thank you. After a moment or two of silence he said, "The correct response to 'thank you' is 'you're welcome'." I was shocked. I knew that was the response. Why didn't I use it? Because I realized 'you're welcome' was rarely used at home. It was expected that as the child I would say 'thank you' but my father rarely if ever said, 'you're welcome'. I realized that when I said 'thank you' and never received a response I always felt like I hadn't done something quite well enough to rate getting a 'you're welcome' reply. In terms of understanding bless-ings, receiving, and gratitude – it was the everyday expressions 'thank you' and 'you're welcome' that got my attention.

I couldn't wait to get home and start trying it out. I started saying 'thank you' whenever the opportunity presented itself and it was usually met with silence. But I kept at it. Instead of saying 'thank you' to me, my father might say something like 'well, good' to which I made a point of responding with 'you're welcome'. I did that at every opportunity I got and after some time he began to say 'thank you' every now and then and a couple of times 'you're welcome' escaped his lips.

It was a wonderful game for me because I understood what it was about. I really did mean 'thank you' when I said it and when 'you're welcome' was returned it was so exciting. When my father said 'thank you' and I got to say 'you're welcome' I felt so good. It was like I had just done the best thing in the world for somebody else. It reminded me of the word Namasté that we used in yoga class – the God in me recognizes and honors the God in you. I came to understand that for me resistance begins to melt in front of 'thank you' and it's a puddle after 'you're welcome'.

Transit Toss

All right – think

Why did this happen?

Is this just another example of my usual routine – two steps forward, three back?

How could that be? Have I learned nothing?

Here I am lying in bed and it's the start of week number two.

I cannot believe the pain I am in.

I cannot even begin to consider getting out of bed and back into my wheelchair.

Ha. Now there's a thought.

I would never have believed that the idea of getting back into my wheelchair would be an improvement in my life.

That's a good one...

I had just gotten on the bus on my scooter headed home from having met my parents for coffee. I was living in the co-op now and my parents had their own apartment a block away from the condo we shared for seven years. Since the spring I had been riding Edmonton's low floor buses and LRT all over the city. My scooter and public transportation brought luscious independence back into my life. I created daily adventures for myself, rediscovering places I hadn't been to in a long time and saw new places I'd only heard about.

It was just before Thanksgiving and I met my parents for coffee at a restaurant to discuss plans for the upcoming weekend. My brother and his family were coming to Edmonton for the Thanksgiving holiday. They were coming from their home in southern Alberta. It was going to be the first time I met my niece. She was fifteen months old, walking and talking, but I hadn't met her yet. It was too difficult for me to travel to their home. My parents had seen her and we had pictures but I was so looking forward to meeting her in person for the first time.

After we discussed our plans for the weekend I got on the bus headed home. I had been on this bus route many times before traveling between the co-op where I lived and my parents' apartment. It was a route I knew well and it only took ten minutes to get between both places. I gave the bus driver my ticket and got the scooter parked on the right side of the bus. There was a fellow sitting in the first row of seats behind me. The three-seater bench directly opposite me on the left side of the bus had been turned up against the wall. There was a couple sitting in the first row of seats facing forward behind that.

I looked up at the rear view mirror and saw the driver, a young East Indian man, having an animated conversation all by himself. No one was near him and my first thought was "Oh my, we have a crazy driver on the bus." I made note of the number of the bus just in case somebody wanted to know exactly which bus the crazy driver was on. Then I thought maybe he was on a cell phone and I hadn't noticed the earpiece when I boarded.

I got on the bus at the corner of Jasper and 116th Street. We headed south along 116th Street and then turned west on to Victoria Park Hill. The bus picked up speed going down the hill, with our driver laughing and talking to whomever it was he was imagining.

At the bottom of the hill there were two turns the bus had to make, one to the left and the second to the right as it made its approach on to Groat Bridge. The bus didn't slow down. It made the first swing to the left and picked up speed. The second swing to the right was coming up. When the bus got on the bridge it had to flow with traffic coming on its left side. I thought it would slow down a bit to do the merge but it didn't. Instead the bus accelerated. It swung hard right. The momentum threw me and the scooter across the bus slamming my head into the left side wall and twisting my neck so my chin was jammed into the base of my throat. The left side of my skull was wedged against my shoulder and my left arm was trapped against the wall. I was on my side, my left hip ground into the floorboards and the scooter had landed on my lower right leg. I was pinned. I couldn't move and every part of me stabbed with pain.

I laid there in stunned shock while my brain madly ran through a checklist of body parts. Could I move? What hurt? What hurt more? I was flaming angry and in tears.

That %#$* idiot driver. Who did he think he was? Mario Andretti?! Is this how he got his jollies? Drive a great big bus way too fast down a long hill and then – could he make those tires squeal? Swing one time to the left and haul on that steering wheel. Swing one more time to the right. Stand on the accelerator. Scare the hell out of oncoming traffic. Yeehaw.

He saw me get on the bus. Did he think I was riding the scooter just for show? Did he not think that *maybe* he should drive with a little bit more *care and attention* because he had a passenger on a scooter parked right at the front of the bus? It wasn't like I was hiding.

Besides toss-the-crip, did he also play stop-the-bus-fast-and-see-if-the-old-lady-in-the-aisle-falls-down? Who was this bricks-for-brains-twit and how did he get this job? I was livid. If I could've gotten up and screamed obscenities in his face, I would've done it.

My twisted head, neck and shoulder were pasted to the left wall of the bus while the rest of me laid on the floor under the scooter in front of the couple in the first row of seats facing forward behind the driver. The woman identified herself as Gayle. She took my hand and tried to calm me. She said an ambulance had been called. I opened my eyes long enough to see a man talking on a cell phone. I don't think he was the driver but maybe he was. I closed my eyes and didn't open them again.

When the ambulance arrived a female paramedic introduced herself as Janice – or was that Janet? She wanted to know where it hurt. My brain was still scrambling through body parts assessing damages. I wanted to say it all hurt but she kept asking for specifics. She pressed the back of my neck with her fingers and said, "Does that hurt?" Yes. Every place she touched hurt.

I was able to give Janice-Janet instructions about where to get my ID and Blue Cross card in my fanny pack. She started asking me questions that I realized were just to see if my brains were working right. She asked me how old I was. I said fifty-two but my internal voice immediately questioned my response. Was I fifty-two? Do the math I told myself. I was born in 1953. It's now 2005. Three from five is two and five from ten is five. That's fifty-two. There I was doing the math and doing it correctly but not trusting the answer. Maybe the number surprised me. Maybe I didn't think of myself as fifty-two. Was I really that old? Wow...

I could hear there was some discussion about the ambulance. Janice-Janet asked me if I could get off the bus on my own. Did she mean walk I asked her? Yes, she said. No, I answered calmly but there were questions swirling in my head like "What do you think the scooter's for? Do you think I get a cut rate on bus fares if I show up on the scooter working that sympathy angle? No, I answered calmly. I have multiple sclerosis. I let the part about not being able to walk dangle in mid-air hoping the paramedic would be able to make the association between scooter and multiple sclerosis. She asked if I could move. No, I answered calmly but inside my head I was screaming *"I'm smashed up against the side of a bus."* Right, she said and then instructed, "We'll have to get her off on a backboard."

The bus was stopped on the bridge and there was no room for the ambulance to pull up alongside and get me off on a backboard. The bus moved across the bridge to the entrance of Hawrelak Park where there was more room for the paramedics to manoeuvre. When they shifted me on to the backboard I know I made noise. My eyes were still closed and the pain was excruciating especially when they put the collar around my neck. They strapped my body and taped my head to the board to further ensure no movement. Then they slid me off the bus and into the ambulance.

We weren't far from the University of Alberta Hospital so that's where they took me. I heard something being said about x-rays and I thought to myself, "Good God, how are we going to do this?" They took me and the backboard out of the ambulance on to a gurney and wheeled me into a large bay near where the ambulance had parked. They removed the straps, peeled the tape off my head, removed the collar and slid the board out from under me.

The conversation between a male and female technician and the sounds of some kind of machine moving along an overhead track made it clear that I didn't have to go to the x-ray machine. The x-ray machine was moving over and around me.

Well, check this out.

The technicians took a number of x-rays, some areas from different angles, and I didn't have to move at all. I started to relax for the first time. I also started to feel even more pain concentrated in certain areas. Maybe it was because I was relaxing that I was more available to feel the pain. I complained about my left hip and another x-ray was taken of that.

The emergency room doctor came by and started moving my left arm around. He said my shoulder wasn't dislocated. The collar bone wasn't broken. The male technician told him no broken bones were showing up on any of the x-rays.

Seriously?

I couldn't believe it. Neither could the doctor. I had repeatedly told the paramedics that I not only had multiple sclerosis but I also had osteoporosis. When the emergency room doctor made it official and told me there were no broken bones I said again I have multiple sclerosis and osteoporosis. He said it was amazing but there were no broken bones.

The female x-ray technician said that a man from Edmonton Transit had brought my scooter to the emergency ward and he wanted to know what my name and phone number were. She said they weren't allowed to give him that information without my permission. I said they could definitely give him my name and phone number. I expected to be hearing from Edmonton Transit in the very near future.

I was wheeled into the emergency room area and parked by the nurses' desk beside my scooter. The scooter didn't look any the worse for wear, which I was pleased to see. I asked the male nurse if there was a phone I could use. I told him my cell phone was in my fanny pack but I didn't know if using cell phones was allowed in that area. He got a cell phone for me and I called Dan. I told him what had happened and where I was. I was only a few blocks from the co-op so I asked him if he would walk me home if I could get on the scooter. I wanted to make sure I got home safe and sound and I thought after the jolt I had just taken I could use some company. He said yes, he'd be right there. Then I called my parents. I told them what had happened, where I was, that there were no broken bones, and Dan was on his way. They said they would meet me at my apartment.

While I was waiting for Dan to arrive, I listened to the male nurse tell the other nurses about his adventure hunting deer with a bow and arrow. I was chuckling to myself because Dan had taught himself to shoot a bow and arrow with the idea of hunting for deer. The nurses' desk got a call that Dan was in the waiting room looking for me. She gave directions to where I could be found and a few minutes later Dan came into view. What a welcome sight he was.

The male nurse came by with a little paper cup holding three small white pills for me to take for the pain. I said, "I'm sorry, but I was eavesdropping on your story." I looked at him and introduced Dan by saying, "He hunts deer with a bow and arrow." Their conversation was immediately off and running. Then the emergency room doctor came by and said I was probably going to be "pretty sore for a couple of days." He said I was welcome to spend the night in the hospital but the only bed they could give me would be in the emergency ward. Dan thought I should stay but if I stayed I didn't think I would get much rest. The advantages of going home were that there was staff twenty-four hours a day and I would be in my own bed. Dan tried to encourage me to stay in the hospital but I was determined to get home.

The doctor's remark that I was going to be pretty sore for the next couple of days made me think I should get a catheter while I was in the hospital. Getting in and out of the washroom was enough of an exercise for me normally with the MS but if I was going to be this sore for a couple of days that would make using the bathroom a painful challenge. Better to minimize that anguish. I thought it would be best if I could just stay in bed and a catheter would allow me to do that.

When that request had been seen to, I asked Dan and the male nurse if they could help me get on the scooter. One picked me up under the arms and the other picked up my feet. The transfer hurt so much it took my breath away but there was no getting around it if I wanted to go home. While the nurses were helping me get my jacket on, my parents phoned from my apartment where they were waiting for us. I told them Dan and I were on our way.

Getting Home

Dan and I covered the three blocks back to where I lived very slowly. He walked beside me and I rode my scooter hoping not to hit too many bumps on the sidewalk. I was a veritable Chatty Cathy doll describing what had happened. I think it was a combination of shock and pain killers. Dan declared, "Lawsuit!" I said I would charge the city big bucks and take him and his wife to dinner in the city of their choice. We laughed.

When we got back to my place Dan pressed the elevator button and said he knew this was going to happen. By that he meant he knew this accident was going to happen. Why he said that I don't know. Maybe he didn't like the way I drove my scooter. Maybe he figured riding public transit on a scooter was risky business. It doesn't matter how he knew. I just wish he had told me in time so I didn't get on that bus.

When we got to the apartment my parents were there. Dan got me off the scooter and back into my wheelchair in one lift. I knew it would hurt. I warned him before he picked me up I would probably scream but he was not to pay attention to that. I had to get back into my wheelchair. He picked me up ever so gently. It hurt. I hollered. He left.

My mother made some food for me which was great because it was now 9 p.m. and I hadn't eaten anything since the coffee I had when I met them in the afternoon. I was hungry and still talkative and cheery. Good painkillers. When I was done eating I called downstairs to the office and asked for some staff assistance to get me into bed. My parents left with promises they would call back in the morning to see what else I might need.

Two staff members arrived, picked me up out of the wheelchair and tossed me onto the bed like a sack of potatoes. I hollered again – louder. I was expecting to be picked up and placed with care. Wrong.

They said they would leave word at the office for the night staff to check on me every three hours and they left. My mother had put a brand-new bottle of extra strength Tylenol on the table beside my bed. Safe and snug under the covers, I slept and that is where I stayed for the next two weeks.

Aftermath

The doctor's remark that I was going to be pretty sore for the next couple of days was the understatement of the year.

The next morning I awoke in agony. Not only was every body part in pain but all of those parts combined didn't hurt as much as my insides. It felt like every internal organ I had was sitting just below my throat. I found it hard to swallow the smallest sip of water never mind the Tylenol I was also trying to get down with it. I tried to eat a bit of toast but that was virtually impossible. I knew I needed food and water and I also needed that Tylenol but I was having so much trouble swallowing. Breathing was alright as long as I kept it shallow.

When I couldn't stand it anymore I phoned Dan and begged him for help. He wasn't exactly enthusiastic about doing a treatment for me because he explained all of my soft tissue would be so swollen he didn't know what relief he could give me. I begged and he came over that afternoon with his daughter. She assisted with the treatment by monitoring the cranial plates on my skull giving Dan feedback while he assessed the internal damage done by the accident.

I was right about my insides hurting. Dan explained that flying through the air and stopping suddenly when my head slammed against the left bus wall caused all of my internal organs to shift from free-floating to impact. They were indeed sitting jammed together below my throat.

With his skill at therapeutic touch and knowledge of energy systems Dan managed to move my diaphragm almost back into the position it should occupy. Giving me that bit of space was a huge relief. It meant that the other organs could begin to relax and move back into their positions in their own time. His daughter's feedback letting Dan know how I was reacting to his treatment in a clear coherent manner made it possible for him to do his work without having to translate my groans. After his visit I was able to drink and eat which were absolutely essential for me to recover.

Thank God I know Dan and thank God he helps me.

I had been so looking forward to the weekend and my brother and his family's visit that when the accident happened I thought I might miss out on seeing them completely. That upset me almost as much as the accident. But the weekend was saved when my parents and my brother and sister-in-law came over with the kids both Friday and Saturday nights. They also brought doggy bags from the two dinners they ate at my parents' place. So not only did I get to see them and meet my niece for the first time, I also got to eat my mother's Thanksgiving turkey, too. The combination of Dan and Mum is what I call a winning team.

The night staff checked me every three hours. They would help me change position by rolling me onto my side and stuffing pillows at my back to keep me in place or they would remove the pillows letting me lie flat on my back. They alternated giving me Advil and Tylenol. One reduced the swelling and the other reduced the pain. They looked after my personal care needs, kept the apartment functioning and worked with my parents who came in to restock the larder and make meals. The staff also got me a shoebox that they filled with all my vitamin bottles and three water bottles that they filled with water, cranberry juice, and cold green tea. That was great. A friend in the building who was also wheelchair-bound loaned me a foam pillow in the shape of a triangle that supported my back and allowed me to lift my head enough so I could sort of sit up and eat. Another staff member dragged my TV, VCR, and DVD player into the bedroom and hooked it all up so that I could at least watch movies even though I couldn't get television reception. The friend who loaned me the triangle-shaped pillow also gave me some of his DVD's so I wouldn't get bored watching the same movies all the time.

And that was the routine for two straight weeks. Slowly but surely I weaned myself off the Advil and Tylenol but the lingering pain meant I didn't even try to get into the wheelchair until the end of the second week.

What Was That About...?

I was lying in bed looking out the window at the apartment building across the back alley. It looked like a good day. The sky was clear and blue and the sun was reflecting off the other apartment building's windows. It was the start of my second week in bed. I still hurt but I must be feeling better because I was looking at what kind of day it was instead of wondering how long until my next Tylenol.

When one of the staff was making lunch for me earlier, she commented that I was lucky I hadn't broken my leg in the accident. Boy, I thought, she was right about that.

Wait a minute. What was I thinking?

I'd already spent one week in bed in dire pain completely dependent on others. I didn't break my leg or collarbone or dislocate my shoulder. I could've fractured my skull the way I hit the side wall of that bus but instead of breaking bones what I got was a full body whiplash from hell. Why didn't I break something? It was quiet in the apartment. I wasn't expecting anybody for awhile so I lay there pondering the questions floating through my mind, wondering about the answers, enjoying uninterrupted contemplation.

And then it happened. An answer came to me. It was the martyrdom. I had released the belief in martyrdom. Getting tossed on the bus was an excuse, a diversion the Universe had created so I would have a reason to lie in bed and let my body do what it had to do to complete the release. The release was going to hurt like hell because the belief in martyrdom was embedded in every single cell. Somewhere along the line I had given myself permission to wrench the martyrdom belief system from every cell at exactly the same time, the moment of impact when my head smashed into the side wall on that bus. Now I had a reason to lie in bed and rest all those millions of cells so they could adjust to life without martyrdom and heal anew.

When that thought came to me, it was the answer and it was perfectly correct. I knew it. It sounded like science fiction but I knew it was right. I felt so relieved. I didn't hurt any less but now I was more relaxed and receptive to the pain because I understood why I had it. I released the belief in martyrdom. I released the martyrdom. Gonzo. I wasn't thinking "now what" and flinching for the next cosmic hit. I was relaxed and receptive to whatever new stuff was coming. I had nothing to fear. I must be ready for whatever new stuff was headed my way otherwise I wouldn't have been tossed on the bus.

As I thought about it more, it crossed my mind that maybe I could've accomplished the release without having to hurt so much. Did I have to get tossed on a bus? That was a bit dramatic being transferred to an ambulance strapped to a backboard. Well, maybe it was the way I had to do it. Maybe I believed that the only way to get rid of centuries-old-genetic-belief-in-Catholic-inspired-martyrdom was to throttle it out of me. No doubt there are better ways to do these things. Maybe I could have conceived of life without that belief and it would have simply vanished, no fuss no muss. Maybe I could have gently meditated my way to eliminating it from my thoughts. But maybe I wasn't spiritually evolved enough to release martyrdom simply and gently. Maybe I'm evolved enough to identify the belief, recognize its depth and be receptive to letting it go but I'm not spiritually evolved enough to do it painlessly or without drama. Maybe I didn't understand that I could have just let it go. Maybe on some level I thought releasing martyrdom was a big deal and should be experienced as an event. Maybe the Universe orchestrated the bus accident and then gave me this moment of quiet contemplation to wonder at its perfection. I unloaded three hundred and fifty-six years of belief in martyrdom from a 17th century farm on Île d'Orléans to trendy Whyte Avenue in Edmonton and I didn't break a single bone doing it..

God is good.

You should be Dead

Dan said it would take about two months for the swelling to leave the soft tissue and then it would be the right time to work on any physical issues that might need to be addressed. So two months after I was tossed on the bus, I called Kevin and asked if he could check me out for damages I might have sustained.

There was no way I could get to the basement clinic so Kevin came to my apartment, thank goodness. He sat on the couch, paperwork on his lap, conducting the interview while I sat in my wheelchair. He asked detailed questions about the accident and made notes of my answers on one side of a piece of paper. On the other side, there was the diagram of a body that he marked with additional notes. When he had finished conducting the interview he came over to where I was sitting in my wheelchair.

Moving both of his hands from place to place around my skull he asked me to describe again exactly how my head had hit the side wall of the bus. I told him what I remembered and when I was done he said, "No, that's not how you hit." That surprised me. Then he lightly moved my head as he described how the damage on my skull indicated the way I hit the wall of the bus. Ever so carefully, he turned my head to one side, moved my chin down and then twisted my neck to where it would have stopped jammed against the wall of the bus and my left shoulder. "That's it," I said. "That's exactly what it felt like." I was amazed at how accurate he was and how all the feelings and stresses immediately returned to my head and neck with his gentle manipulation.

He checked out my shoulders, collarbone, arms, rib cage, spine, hip, legs, knees, right down to my toes. When he was done he went back to my skull and my neck and said, "You should be dead. You should have broken your neck." Just like that. A simple statement. I was shocked. I would never have expected him to speak so bluntly. He went back and forth between making notes on his information sheet, marking the diagram on the back and examining me in various spots a second time. Before he left that day he made the same statement, that I should be dead, I should have broken my neck three more times.

We worked gradually over the next five months realigning muscle and bone from the top of my head to my feet. We would work on an area and then let two or three weeks pass before our next session. The time in between treatments allowed my body to assimilate the adjustments Kevin had done. During those five months he said I should be dead, I should have broken my neck twice more for a total of six times from the first session. He used the word "miraculous" on four occasions. I counted because I was astounded at how frankly he made the remarks.

Over the next few years I referred a couple of people I knew to Kevin for chiropractic care. On their first visits when he read my name on the referral line of their information sheets, both people reported his comment was, "She should be dead. She should have broken her neck."

But I didn't and I wasn't. That wasn't why the accident happened. It wasn't that I got lucky and survived with only soft tissue injuries, as serious as they were. It was about letting go of a belief I had in martyrdom. I believed it was genetic, in every cell in my body. I believed if I was going to change that and let it go, it was going to hurt. I believe the Universe created the bus accident so I could lie in bed for two weeks in terrific pain and let go of the martyrdom the way I thought I had to. It probably didn't have to happen that way at all. Maybe I could have released it with a good sneeze. In my next life, I'll know better.

The Volunteer

I arrived at the clinic in the middle of a lively discussion between Kevin and Dan. "Are you a victim or a volunteer?" they called out to me. "A victim," I shouted back. They broke up laughing. "That's why I keep coming back," I said. After all the work we had done, I knew a negative word like 'victim' would be the wrong answer. Still chuckling, Kevin ushered his next patient into his office and I followed Dan into his for our appointment. By the time I got home after the session, Dan had already e-mailed a piece his wife had written on the subject of victims and volunteers. I thought it was terrific because it spoke to me about where I was in understanding choices at that point in time and it continues to speak to me. This is what she wrote:

"What is the opposite of a victim? It's a Volunteer. Volunteers make choices. Their choices allow them to do what they must in order to be true to themselves. They take responsibility for all aspects of their lives.

A victim is powerless, living life at the whim of shifting breezes, bemoaning his fate, blaming others for his chaotic circumstances.

Choice is an element of freewill. A Volunteer uses freewill to fuel his creativity and add variety to the choices he can make. A Volunteer takes control. The choices he makes are consistent with who he is and what he needs to conduct his life with integrity.

You have freewill and there is always choice. The choices you make are the bricks in the life structure you build while you're here on this earth. Volunteer for your life.

A Soul's purpose is to be more. It learns. It grows. It moves in and out of realities experiencing the lessons they have to offer in universes we can't begin to imagine beyond this veil that clouds our vision. A Soul cannot be less than what it is and it is so much more than what we think.

Mistakes are part of learning. How can we know the difference unless we've "committed" the error? But having experienced a mistake and become aware that we strayed from our path, we have an obligation to make note of where we made that wrong turn. We need to spend time understanding how it came to happen and think about what we can do to change the outcome the next time those circumstances arise.

Mistakes are opportunities to learn, correct, and move forward with new clarity and energy. Each time we ignore an error we have committed against ourselves, the Universe will repeat the situation – a little louder, a little harder – hoping to get our attention. Continuing to be inattentive or brushing aside the experiences, will only lead to larger, more treacherous detours until finally we come to a dead end.

Volunteers listen. Listen to the thoughts you think. Listen to the words you speak. If a stranger stood in front of you thinking those thoughts and speaking those words, would you want to know them? If they asked you to join them for coffee, would you accept, or would you make an excuse and run away as fast as you could?

Volunteers feel. Feelings, twinges, rising emotions – Volunteers pay heed because they know reason doesn't guide with the sureness of a gut reaction. They trust intuition.

Cathy Asselin

Volunteers observe. They take time to watch what is happening around them, and the part they serve in the play. Stepping back for a better view of the larger scene, they don't miss as many jokes.

In the Christian model, when Christ died for our sins was he a martyr? He took full responsibility for his actions and had the ability and the freedom to get out of it. But He didn't. That's a Volunteer."

Segment 10 – You've a Soul for a Compass

In this world there's a whole lot of cold

In this world there's a whole lot of plain

In this world you've a soul for a compass

And a heart for a pair of wings

There's a star on the far horizon

Rising bright in an azure sky

For the rest of the time that you're given

Why walk when you can fly –

high

Mary Chapin Carpenter
Why Walk When you can Fly
from Stones in the Road

Fascinating Science

If a salamander loses its tail, it will grow a new one.

If a live, human donor donates part of his liver to another person who needs a transplant; both the original liver and the donated section will grow to the right size and shape for each of the donor and the recipient.

War veterans who have lost a limb in battle have been known to complain that their missing leg is itchy when it's been gone for years.

Why does the salamander's severed tail grow back? Why do both the donor and transplanted human liver sections grow to be exactly the right size and shape for both the donor and the recipient? Why does the veteran's missing leg itch?

Science can tell us the answer for each of these scenarios but maybe there's something else. Somewhere between a salamander's tail, a human liver transplant and a veteran's missing leg could there be something else we don't understand yet? Maybe there's a 'spiritual blueprint' of how each of us should be physically. Maybe we will eventually learn how to tap into that 'blueprint' to fix severed spinal cords or rebalance brains struggling with Alzheimer's, Parkinson's, or multiple sclerosis. Maybe we can be in touch with that 'spiritual blueprint' throughout our lives while we need our bodies on this earth. Maybe it's the 'spiritual blueprint' we return to when the lessons for this life's trip to the earth-school are done. It's only one of an infinite array of fascinating possibilities.

The Body's Mandate

There is nothing like the body and the brain. Both are breathtaking masterpieces of engineering, wonders that we may never fully fathom. We may learn a lot about the nuts and bolts of them, but we may never understand all of their mysteries.

I believe the body's mandate is to be healthy.

Like the flame on a candle, no matter which way you turn it, the flame burns upwards. Hold the candle sideways, the flame burns upwards. Point the wick at the floor, the flame burns upwards. No matter how we were born, no matter the illnesses or diseases we have experienced since or the strains, stresses and abuses we've sustained along the way, the body's mandate is to be healthy. As the candle's flame always burns upwards, our body strives for health and balance no matter what the circumstances.

By always trying to maintain health and balance, I believe our body's purpose is to guide, serve and teach us. It is intelligent, vigilant and functions in ways we've only begun to catch sight of. The body knows the difference between fighting an infection by activating fever, or mending a cut by building a protective scab over the wound. How does it know to do these things? How does it know *when* to do these things and which function to activate?

We are composed of billions of cells but they are not all the same cell. From conception, diversity and specialization unfold. Some cells become a heart. Some become bone. Other cells become the delicate web we call the nervous system. How do they know to do that? How do some cells know to become a liver instead of an eyeball? How do they know what their jobs are and how do they know how to do them?

I think the body is astounding. Scientists can give you logical scientific explanations for how or why everything works but for me I think it's magic. What kind of magic directs a single cell to divide and diversify with such variety and complexity that it becomes a human being? And what tells all those diverse and specialized cells to cooperate with each other communicating with the exquisite precision necessary to build a healthy, fully functioning man or woman?

When I was diagnosed with MS I felt my body was betraying me but with time I learned that mentally and emotionally I was the one who was letting *it* down.

A thoughtful man I know commented that he believed the body is the operating manual for our life. When you're not sure what's happening in your life, what is your body telling you? Watch. Feel. It's giving you signals. It's communicating with you, trying to give you messages about what is going on in your life and how it feels about it. Are the thoughts you're thinking positive? Are the emotions you're feeling bringing you hope and peace or upset? Are you tired or are you energized with joy and creativity? Is there room in your day for enthusiasm?

From time to time he speculated we may need minor adjustments, a tune-up now and then that the body can do for us. We sneeze because we are on the verge of getting a cold or we strain our backs because we're not in the right position when we're working hard. Maybe a more serious course correction is required so we seek medical advice. Maybe that course correction is the kind of issue we come to realize is why we are on this earth in this life. We are here to work through and understand it. It's the kind of challenge that demands courage. No matter what is required to keep us moving in the upward progressive movement of life, I believe the body gives us the opportunity to learn and it is our obligation to do so. It's not always fun but then that's the human in me talking.

The Body is self-regulating and has mechanisms capable of handling an astounding amount of stress, strain and change. The problem is we are easily distracted and don't pay attention. Oftentimes we are already way down the road on a serious situation before we pause and look around. Sometimes we are made to stop before we look up. I was stopped and even then I spent a lot of time looking around for something to blame because I couldn't cross the street the way I wanted to. It took a long time before I could sit quietly with the paralysis and begin to understand some of what it was trying to tell me. What I began to understand it was trying to tell me was that I was the only one who was holding me to a standard of false expectations. Nobody and nothing else was. It was just me and I didn't start to even think in those terms until I was stopped – literally.

Sometimes I think MS is a pretty harsh lesson but it was probably the best lesson for me. I have no idea how God would have gotten my attention otherwise. I believe my experience with multiple sclerosis is why I'm here in this lifetime. There could be any number of reasons why it exists in my body – maybe I caught a virus; maybe the water supply in this city is contaminated; maybe there is a weak link in the chain of my genetics that says I was doomed to have this from the get-go. I believe the emotional confusion and grinding negativity of my mental conversations with myself I call the Martyr Heroine, operated for such a long stretch of time that they made some kind of physical breakdown inevitable. My body was fertile ground for whatever other factors might have been involved with the onset of my MS.

Tangled Expectations

I believe I'm here in this life to learn from it and forgive myself for whatever issues I may have brought to its creation. I believe the possibility exists to change it for the better or eliminate it completely from my body. Assistance will come in a therapy or a medical procedure or a pill that will help me physically to right myself. Perhaps I will learn to allow so much joy, contentment and love into my life that there will simply be no reason for the MS to exist anymore in this body. Whatever happens, I want to be in the best possible frame of mind, heart, and body to receive it.

Choices

A disease may manifest similar symptoms from one person to another but the reasons for having the illness in the first place are as unique and distinctly separate as snowflakes. If I think about it, I'll bet I had warnings. There were probably many times when I could have made another choice in my thinking or what I said or in my behaviour. Where did I go off track? Why did I surrender myself to someone or something else? Why did I decide to take some action I knew I didn't want to do? Was I actually aware I was doing something I was uncomfortable with?

It doesn't matter. I can change it later.

When did I give up being the real me? What was I doing when the Universe decided enough was enough and stopped me in my tracks from going where I thought I was headed?

Somewhere rattling around in the back of my mind I knew I had a choice but I didn't know it consciously. I certainly didn't know it emotionally. Consciousness was a gradual dawning. Slowly but surely, with the experiences I kept butting up against, it dawned on me there could be another way to think and another way to do things. I began to understand that I could choose to look after myself and pursue what interested me or I could work against myself. I was perfectly free and able to make different choices. Whenever I made a choice that acknowledged what I really wanted to do, things fell into place and moved forward easily. When I didn't make a good choice, taking it back was messy, time-consuming, energy depleting and filled with frustration and anxiety. Not worth it. I made choices that didn't honor who I was and the Universe felt paralysis was the way to get my attention. It literally made me stop and reconsider the thoughtless patterns I was swirling in. Now was my chance to make things right with myself.

I noticed that if one day was lousy the next day would be better. If I needed to be self-indulgent for a day and be sad then that was okay. I started to give myself permission to feel miserable when I felt miserable. I chose to wallow in my misery because I *knew* the next day would be better. I also noticed the wallowing time got shorter, like a mud puddle drying in the sun got smaller. The mud puddle was still there. It hadn't dried up completely but it wasn't the mud-slide that used to bury me.

Each day I peeled back the layers of what was happening to me. Sometimes it was tedious trying to figure it out and sometimes I understood immediately and peeled back that layer with a flourish. Sometimes it hurt and sometimes it was the definition of scary but always there were gifts. I didn't see the gifts at first because I was too busy looking the other way. When I did see them, they took my breath away because I didn't see them coming.

One of those gifts was giving me credit for good choices I *had* made. I couldn't go back to the beginning of my life but I could go back to my diagnosis. It was a great decision to drive out of the parking lot at that first neurologist's office and choose never to go back. It was a great decision to meet Dan the first time, although perhaps not wise to go to a building I had never been to before to meet a man I didn't know but I chose to trust my instincts and the sound of his voice. The second half of this life started with great decisions and good choices.

The Soul's Mandate

In grade school, I was taught that each of us has a soul and it is a piece of God. I liked that story so I decided it was true. Today, I believe that each soul is a single spark of the energy I call God. I think of the soul as God's twinkle. Looking at the sky on a clear night with all the stars above is what I imagine God sees when He looks at all the souls in the universe.

I believe the soul's mandate is to be more.

I think each soul is perpetually evolving at its own rate and in its own time. I believe the soul becomes more by learning. It grows through experience and the learning that comes with it. I believe each of us sets up the parameters for learning that will enable us to grow and be more with every lifetime we live. I believe we set up the time, experiences, circumstances, people we interact with, and the families we are born into. We don't know the outcome of each lifetime because on this Earth the element of free will is at play. When the life has been completed for that go-round, I believe we return to the energy that is God. Our latest life experiences make us more, which makes God more. After a lifetime, I believe we take as much time as we want to rest and evaluate the life we have just concluded. We play and work at those activities that interest us and contribute to the God-Energy until we are ready to experience another life. When we are ready, we design a life that will give us the best learning for further growth.

I believe Earth is only one of the situations where a soul can go to learn and become more through experience. Earth must be a popular learning destination because it has an intriguing combination of parameters. It's three dimensional, with polarities, and offers a blending of experiences that are physical, mental, spiritual and emotional. I believe we choose the circumstances of our life on Earth while we are with the God-Energy before we get here. We choose the other souls we will interact with and we agree with each other before we begin the story, what it is each of us is trying to learn or understand.

We set it up but when we arrive here we have no memory of where we came from. We're blind, deaf and dumb about what we truly are. We wander around bumping into things and each other, coming to conclusions that nine times out of ten may not be quite right but I believe we are guided by a spiritual instinct that is like a half remembered song. We have cosmic intuition, the Soul's whisper, and we have free will. We can make choices and change our minds. We have consciousness that we can awaken if we so choose. Lives spent on this planet are the expressions of the choices we make, the free will we exercise while we are here learning.

Like surviving a wild crazy ride at an amusement park, when the ride is over and we've caught our breath from screaming and laughing, sometimes we want to go back and do it again. When the exhibition is over, we can't wait for the midway to come back to town next year. So, too, I believe we can have more than one lifetime be it on Earth or some other situation in the universe. Who knows what possibilities are out there?

I believe the purpose of having a life experience on Earth is just that – to have the experience, to learn, and be more. When we're here stumbling around, what we're looking for is the path Home, back to the God-Energy whether we understand it that way or not. We want to arrive Home with a wealth of new experience about what we are as sparks of God that will propel us into more learning on or off this planet. We have an insatiable desire to be more.

Our Sun is one of billions of stars in a spiral galaxy we call the Milky Way. It is estimated that there are billions of galaxies in this universe. Scientists believe the universe is expanding. If individual souls go out into the universe to have experiences that provide learning so they become more, then it makes sense that the universe is expanding. It has also been theorized that there could be other self-contained universes that aren't aware of each other

I believe there are an infinite number of ways for a Soul to experience learning. There are "realities" of one dimension, two dimensions, and dimensions we cannot grasp. There is life, work, and purpose whether we are living on this planet or not.

How could there *not* be life on other planets, in other galaxies and other universes? How great is this God-Energy, this Force, All-That-Is, He/She, the Source, Creator – whatever you call it – how great is that?

Illness may be part of the plan my Soul decided on before I entered this life. Illness may provide the best lessons for the evolution of my spirit at this time. It may be how I leave this physical lifetime or it may be a warning shot, a chance to re-create myself while I'm here.

The First Word

In the days before pre-school and pre-pre-school, when kindergarten was a new concept, my mother asked me if I would like to go to kindergarten. I asked her what that was and she said it was a kind of school that I could go to before I went to grade one. I asked her if I had to go to grade one and she said yes. I asked her if I had to go to kindergarten and she said no. I decided on the spot I didn't want to go to kindergarten because once I went to school that's what I would be doing for a very, very long time. It was important to me to keep as much free time in my life for as long as I could.

So when I got to grade one I didn't know how to read, I didn't know the alphabet and I didn't know how to write. At the time, that was the case with most kids starting school. Not like kids today who go to all those pre-pre-schools and learn all those things before they start grade one and they better know all those things before they go through the doors of an elementary school because the world is moving so much faster now.

In grade one we learned the alphabet. We learned each new letter, learned the order they came in and learned how to print them.

Penmanship was critical. We printed pages and pages of each letter with our brand new HB pencils in fresh lined copybooks also known as scribblers.

We learned there were two kinds of alphabet. We printed the alphabet in small letters. We printed the alphabet in capital letters. I loved the smell of new paper and owning pencils sharpened to points and having a Pink Pearl eraser. We weren't allowed to have pens. We were too young. We weren't allowed to have pens until grade four. In grade four we got to use straight pens with nibs – the metal detachable point you inserted into the straight pen, which was a fancy stick really. We had bottles of ink in our choice of colors – black or blue. The bottles sat in the ink well holes cut into the top of our wooden desks. The use of fountain pens with removable cartridges in peacock green ink was controversial. We weren't to use ballpoint pens until we got to high school.

I really enjoyed learning the alphabet – all these letters, filling up pages of the scribbler – I loved learning it. Aside from learning each of the letters, we also learned a sound that came with each character. "A" sounded like this; "W" sounded like that. Letters had sounds. *Fascinating.*

And then one day the teacher told us to open our copybooks to a new page and at the top of the page we were to write the letter "m" and then the letter "e". I did that very precisely. And then she said to sound it out. Well, there was *mmm* for the "m" and *eee* for the "e".

Mmm for the "m". Eee for the "e".

Mmm for "m". Eee for "e".

Mmm. Eee.

MmmEee.

Me. It's Me.

It's a *word* the teacher said. Understanding ripped through my brain like a sparkler on steroids. It was *spelling* she explained. She said if I put all those letters and sounds together I could make words. If I could make words, I could read. It felt like someone had cracked open my head to let the light pour in. I could *read*. I could read *anything* because I knew all the sounds for all of the letters. As if that wasn't enough, she said I could write – anything I wanted to.

I could write – *my Name.*

My imagination sizzled and my heart melted. It wasn't only letters and words. It was stories. It was books. What power was created when a simple two-letter word made the alphabet, sounds, spelling, reading and writing fall into place in one dizzying thud of comprehension. It was personal, eloquent and profound.

I did write stories, silly little simplistic stories that had characters and dialogue and my wonderful mother with patience and strong fingers, typed them for me on an old Underwood typewriter we had. I could watch each heavy metal button my mother pressed rise from the center of the machine and strike the cloth ribbon against the paper as it curved up over the roller. When my mother finished typing, she would hand me a crisp white page with actual typewriter printing on it. It was my story officially printed. A story I had imagined and printed by hand on a lined pad of paper could actually go into production.

Writing a story meant I had to search for just the right words. I remember asking my mother one time how to spell *samater*. When she asked me what I meant, I said that I wanted this person in the story to ask *'what samater'*. It was great when she typed it out because I could actually see it – 'What's the matter?' These are good things to know and I tried not to make the same mistake twice.

Years later when I saw the movie *The Miracle Worker,* I watched Anne Bancroft as Annie Sullivan pump water from a well over Patty Duke's hand as she portrayed Helen Keller. At the same time as the water washed over Helen's hand, Annie made the sign language hand shapes for the word "water" in Helen's palm. I knew what "water" must have felt like for that blind deaf girl to finally connect with the outside world. It was *magic.*

I Am

It has taken me all of my life to get from *Me* to *I am* but maybe that's the way it's supposed to be. So I can report with confidence: I got there. Does that mean that's the end of the story, I've crossed the finish line and there are no more new horizons ahead? Absolutely not. It means it's a new beginning, another level, the next stage, and with it new adventures, new challenges and more fun.

There was a statement I heard that I liked but I wasn't sure which way I liked it best. The statement was *I Am becoming that which I Am* – or did I like it better to say – *I Am that which I Am becoming*? I gave it some thought and said both statements out loud a couple of times so I could hear what they sounded like. I decided I liked saying the statement *I Am that which I Am becoming*. I like hearing it said that way because it says I'm still evolving. To say 'I Am becoming that which I Am' sounds like I've arrived, it's finished, I'm done. There's nowhere else to go. I like the idea that there's more to come so to say I was still *becoming,* whatever that's going to be, appeals to me because there's no conclusion.

Cathy Asselin

I have travelled from *Me* to *I Am*. As *Me* I have grown from being the center of a finite world to recognizing that *I Am* an ever-evolving spark of God in a space continuum so vast it is more than I will ever know sitting on this planet, but sitting on this planet is a significant exploit in an infinite adventure.

Segment 11 – Creating Oneself Endlessly

To exist is to change,

to change is to mature,

to mature is to go on

creating oneself endlessly.

Henri Bergson

Keep Breathing

I did believe that God doesn't play dice. I did believe the universe is not the result of uncontrolled chaos. I did believe everything happens for a reason even if we don't understand why at this moment. I did believe there are no coincidences. I believed those things but at the same time I held these beliefs at arms' length. I believed them but I operated as if they really didn't have anything to do with my life. I reacted to my MS diagnosis like God was out to get me, the universe was a dangerous place, there was no rhyme or reason to having MS and coincidences only happened when circumstances lined up in a crapshoot, like for a lottery win, and those only happened to other people.

I thought I was being proactive when I called the local chapter of the MS Society and got their information package for the 'newly diagnosed'. When I pulled the papers out of the envelope the first page was pink and had the word "pain" written across the top in big, black, block letters. I shoved the papers back in the envelope and I should've tossed it out right then but I read the package later.

Mistake.

When I did read it, I believed all the miserable possibilities it detailed. Then I bolted as far and as fast as fear could take me. When I looked around at where I was, Dan and Kevin were there gently coaxing me down from the treetop.

Days when I was upset, consumed with fatigue, and my thoughts were twisted and scrambled, I could see no light at the end of the tunnel. I didn't know which way was up most times. When I yelled at God and He did something nice for me almost immediately that just added to my frustration. It also didn't help being told I should accept what was happening to me. That was like throwing gasoline on a fire. There was no way I was going to say it's all right if I'm too tired to work properly and I can't do my job anymore. It wasn't okay with me if I couldn't drive and I had to give up my car or I didn't mind if I couldn't walk. And hey, not only did the package say I could look forward to a lifetime of pain but it said I could also go blind. I was supposed to accept all of that as my lot in life?

Let the good times roll.

I didn't accept what was happening to me but with each phase I guess I got used to the gradual changes. I fought against my shifting reality by adapting to it as needed. When my walking was unsteady and unpredictable I used a cane. That meant I could keep working. The walking poles were a treat because I stood straight, I could go up and down stairs and I could look at someone face to face. I met the nicest people using the walking poles and a lot of good men. When they could be helpful and open a door for me, they always gave me the feeling that I had just made their day. Then came the wheelchair and I adapted because it made getting around easier and I could still do some chores. By responding to my changing circumstances, I inadvertently accepted them.

Along the way I started to pay attention to my life and what was happening around me thanks to spending so much time with Dan and Kevin. I listened and heard what they said. Time after time, no matter how distressed and confused I was, they patiently got me pointed in the right direction. It took years and a lot of tissues but the discoveries I made and the laughter we had outweighed the dark patches. The diagnosis scared me so badly I had to reach outside of myself and that was good. Dan and Kevin taught me to trust, first them and then they turned my thinking around so I could start trusting myself. Life got better when I incorporated the lesson that it was okay to speak up and ask for what I wanted, not just for what I needed. I was still in a wheelchair but with adjustments to my attitude and diet, my energy and stamina improved and the MS stabilized.

I began to observe myself. I saw the effect my thoughts had on how my day went. I started to see the bread crumbs. I felt like I was being led and there was help all around me even if sometimes I didn't think it was offered the way I expected. In fact, if I got my expectations out of the way I could be delightfully surprised. Turning fifty was a delightful surprise.

I'm grateful I got slammed against the side of that bus. Lying in bed for two weeks gave me the opportunity and the time to put a lot of my learning together. I don't know that I came to all the right conclusions but I do think the transit toss lined me up for the next set of personal understandings I had and made peace for me with other issues like how I felt about my father.

My father passed away with lung cancer nine months after the bus accident. When he got the news of the cancer, he went into an immediate flurry of activity making his final arrangements and making sure Mum and I would be set up after he was gone. We sold the condo and my parents moved into a seniors' apartment building one block away. I moved to a co-op where I had put in an application a year before. The co-op also had services for someone like me who was disabled and needed extra help with their daily activities. When the dust settled, it seemed like my father relaxed. I remember commenting to Dan how nice my father was and how much I was enjoying his company. That was not something I would have said about him before the cancer.

When we were living together in the condo my parents went out twice sometimes three times a day on various errands. They kept up that routine after they moved to the seniors' apartment only they added chemo and radiation treatments to their outings. My father got up every morning, shaved and dressed before they went out to see what was going on in the city. My mother said one day after they came home from errands, my father parked the car, said 'that's it' and walked away. Six weeks later he was gone.

The last three weeks of his life he spent in the hospital in palliative care. I saw him every day. Usually, my mother was at the hospital in the morning and I would get there on my scooter in the afternoon. When I arrived, she would go for lunch or take a walk or go for coffee with friends. When she came back for my father's dinner service, I went home for mine.

When my father was still at home, he couldn't bend down to give me a kiss with 'hello' because the cancer had gotten into his bones and bending was too painful for him. Sitting in the wheelchair or on the scooter I couldn't reach up high enough to kiss him on the cheek either so we took to holding each other's hands as our sign of affection. The first time I came into his hospital room after he checked into the palliative ward, he held his hand out to me over the bed rail so I could hold it. I loved that.

Those afternoons when I sat on my scooter beside his bed while he slept, I would close my eyes and think thoughts to him. I believed some part of his being would get my thoughts so I could tell him things. In silent conversations I told him everything I wanted to say from how miserable he could be, to issues I thought he was absolutely wrong about, to 'I love you'. For me, those afternoon meditations created forgiveness and appreciation for the man my father was and after he died I could smile and say how lucky I was to have had so much time with him.

I live a pretty normal life except my aspirations to appear on *Dancing with the Stars* have had to be temporarily shelved. I see friends and family regularly. They keep me laughing and interested in life. I go to movies, concerts and sites of interest around town. I do my best to stay away from negative people or those who are avidly interested in sharing the nitty-gritty detail of their ailments and expect me to be just as keen to share mine.

I've removed 'spontaneity' from my vocabulary and replaced it with 'arrangements'. That can be boring but if I look after the details, arrangements can definitely make an event. I am now what they used to call 'high maintenance'. I don't dare travel without lots of extra travel insurance, supplies and/or equipment and I travel with the help of an aide. There are disappointments like when I have to decline an invitation I've received to go some place where access to the location isn't cripple-friendly. There are ways to do most things though like how I've gotten into office buildings through loading docks and underground garages and entered restaurants by going in the back door through the kitchen.

I stay current with the latest news about MS treatments and let my neurologist know I'm interested if something comes up. I don't want to be counted out for one reason or another from being considered for a possible remedy. And I do believe there will be an answer for an effective MS treatment, if not a cure, in my lifetime.

Another movie favourite of mine is *Cast Away*. It has so many great moments but the scene that truly speaks to me happens near the end of the film when Tom Hanks' character, Chuck, is talking to his friend and former work colleague, Stan. Chuck tells Stan that when even his attempt to commit suicide on the island failed, he realized he had power over nothing; there was no way he would ever see his home again and that he would probably die on the island, alone. But that was also the moment he says he knew he had to stay alive. He had to keep breathing. So that's what he did and one day the tide washed two sides of a metal locker on to the beach. He used those two pieces of metal as a sail on a raft he built and the wind lifted the raft with the metal sail and him over the largest waves and out to open sea.

Chuck tells Stan the thought of his girlfriend, Kelly, kept him alive on the island for four years but he had seen her that evening and knew she had moved on with her life. As sad as he was, he knew what he had to do – keep breathing. He knew if he did that, the sun would shine tomorrow and you never knew what the tide was going to bring.

That scene always reminds me that the "tide" has been bringing everything I need for the challenges of this lifetime since the day I was born. The tide brought me my parents and siblings, and even though there have been times when we weren't crazy about each other, we kept breathing and I'm glad we did. When things were at their scariest, Dan and Kevin arrived on shore and got me over the breakers. I have tremendous friends who go back as far as grade one. There are moments from the past that come back to inspire me with lessons about the possibilities for today like my then four-year-old brother's perfect swan dive; or my sister's talent for winning the biggest stuffed animals on the midway at the Calgary Stampede whenever she wanted, as many as she wanted just because she knew she could; or a timely magazine article or a book on my book-shelf that has been there for twenty years. These were some of the bread crumbs leading me back to my path. I didn't see them until I needed to but they were right there when I did. Lying in bed bruised and battered for two weeks I started to see how many bread crumbs there were.

I believe I made all the arrangements for this lifetime before I got here – the people, the circumstances, the challenges and the lessons. If I was the one who put all those pieces together then what did I have to fear? Always there was free choice.

The frustration still flares from time to time but I forgive myself sooner for those crummy moments. I relax more easily and am confident in my belief that something else is on its way, probably something better.

I don't know why my grandfather didn't get sick quarantined on that troop ship for three weeks during the Spanish flu pandemic. I don't know why my father never got chickenpox, measles or mumps when he was a little boy and I don't know why I have multiple sclerosis. At this moment, it's a mystery and I can only speculate. The good news is I didn't experience pain with the MS as advertised on that pink piece of paper and I didn't lose my sight.

I got it back.

Message from Dan

Email received September 2001

I think I am in this work for the adventure. Yes. That is what it is. Why else would I put myself on the line so many times? I'm always stretching things to the limit. This work is like an extreme sport for me. Some people snowboard, jump off cliffs, climb mountains. I work in the clinic.

Getting better is great but the adventure is better. What about you, let's look at it as an extreme sport and getting better is the reward. But the journey is also the reward. I like that.

Resources

Bach, Richard (1979). Illusions – *The Adventures of a Reluctant Messiah.* New York: Dell Publishing Co., Inc.

Boroch, Ann (2007). *Healing Multiple Sclerosis.* Los Angeles: Quintessential Healing, Inc. Publishing.

Dass, Ram with Stephen Levine (1981). Grist for the Mill. Santa Cruz: Bantam New Age Books.

Dyer, Wayne W. (2004) *The Power of Intention.* Carlsbad, CA: Hay House, Inc.

Hay, Louise L. (1988) *Heal Your Body.* Carson, CA.: Hay House, Inc.

Hay, Louise L. (1994) *You Can Heal Your Life.* Carson, CA: Hay House, Inc.

Lipton, Bruce H. (2009) *The Biology of Belief.* Carlsbad, CA: Hay House, Inc.

Ruiz, don Miguel (2001). "The Edifice of the Dream" in *Sixth Sun: A Sixth Sun Foundation Newsletter.* Teotihuacan, Mexico: Sixth Sun Foundation.

And use the power of music. Play your favourite *songs often and loud. Get lost in your imagination singing, dancing, appreciated and grateful. Cheer and be cheered to an inspired beat.*